The Weight Loss
Surgery Workbook

Deciding on Bariatric Surgery,

Preparing for the Procedure, and Changing

Habits for Post-Surgery Success

Doreen A. Samelson, EdD, MSCP

New Harbinger Publications, Inc.

Distributed in Canada by Raincoast Books

Copyright © 2011 by Doreen A. Samelson
       New Harbinger Publications, Inc.
       5674 Shattuck Avenue
       Oakland, CA 94609
       www.newharbinger.com

Cover design by Amy Shoup
Acquired by Melissa Kirk
Edited by Nelda Street

Library of Congress Cataloging-in-Publication Data

Samelson, Doreen A.
  The weight loss surgery workbook : deciding on bariatric surgery, preparing for the procedure, and changing habits for post-surgery success / Doreen A. Samelson ; foreword by Arnold D. Salzberg.
    p. cm.
  Includes bibliographical references.
  ISBN 978-1-57224-899-1 (pbk.) -- ISBN 978-1-57224-900-4 (pdf ebook) 1. Obesity--Surgery--Popular works. 2. Gastrointestinal system--Surgery--Popular works. 3. Weight loss--Popular works. I. Title.
  RD540.S278 2011
  617.4'3--dc22

          2011005852

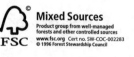

13   13   11

10 9 8 7 6 5 4 3 2 1

First printing

To my daughter, who chose active duty over an easier path; your commitment to military medicine inspires me every day.

To the men in my life; your support and love mean everything.

Contents

Part 1
Making the Decision

Part 2
Preparing for Success by Taking Action

Part 3

Life After Weight Loss Surgery

Acknowledgments

All the patients who came to my office over the years, ready to improve their lives, inspired this book. I'm grateful for each one who chose to share with me her struggles with obesity. These people's bravery and willingness to change have taught me so much. I'm also grateful to Genevieve Fadden, who supports the psychological testing I do with each patient. Without her, my job would be much more difficult.

I'm also grateful to my family, who have supported my work as a medical psychologist and believed in me. And finally, thanks to my fellow California Psychological Association (CPA) members, whose fellowship and support always encourage me.

Foreword

The social, economic, and health costs of morbid obesity have ballooned to epidemic proportions. According to the American Society for Metabolic and Bariatric Surgery (2005), a quarter of the population is obese, and 97 million Americans are overweight. The prevalence of obesity has increased by more than 60 percent in the last ten years. Obesity contributes to three hundred thousand deaths annually, making it second only to smoking as a cause of preventable death. It's a major risk factor for hypertension, type 2 diabetes, cardiac disease, stroke, sleep apnea, osteoarthritis, and many types of cancer. The annual cost of obesity is estimated at $238 billion, of which $33 billion each year is spent on weight loss products. Those suffering from morbid obesity encounter challenges in every facet of life. And to many, it's quite literally a matter of life and death.

Until recently, medical dogma dictated that obesity be managed with medical weight loss programs, appetite suppressants, hypnosis, or hormonal therapy. Surgery was viewed as an extreme measure, to be undertaken only in the direst of circumstances. But most attempts at nonsurgical weight loss are characterized by yo-yo dieting and only short-term weight loss, ultimately leading to an even greater weight gain. In fact, a successful medical weight-loss program is defined as a loss of 10 percent of a patient's excess body weight, or approximately ten pounds in a patient with one hundred excess pounds (Mason et al. 2003). Fewer than 3 percent of people who are morbidly obese can sustain weight loss for one year (ibid.).

As a surgeon performing weight loss surgery, I've seen firsthand how diets fail to produce sustained weight loss, putting patients at additional risk of life-threatening obesity-related medical conditions. Current studies (Robinson 2009) show that the only way sufferers of morbid obesity can lose weight and maintain the weight loss necessary to reverse risk factors is through surgery combined with behavioral changes and nutritional counseling. Further, the current surgical practices to achieve weight loss are safe and effective (ibid.).

But the treatment of morbid obesity and the resolution of obesity-related medical conditions don't begin and end solely in the operating room. While weight loss surgery is a necessary component, significant weight loss requires a multidisciplinary team approach, at the center of which is the patient. The path to success begins preoperatively, with education and behavioral change. Rigorous dietary changes are critical before surgery. After surgery, this commitment must remain the focal point, because the dietary, exercise, and behavioral changes must be maintained for life. With the proper follow-through, loss of upwards of 65 percent of excess body weight can be maintained over ten or more years (Robinson 2009).

Patients suffering from morbid obesity are under unique stressors, requiring empathy, compassion, and support in addition to medical care. Obesity makes every hour of every day more difficult and, quite simply put, removes years from lives. I tell this to the patients coming to be evaluated for surgery so that they may not only understand the gravity of their situation but also come to see the important role each individual must take on his path to recovery, and to instill hope for what is to come. Diabetes will improve and go away, hypertension will resolve, sleep will be more restful, and joints will no longer be painful. Years will be added, lives prolonged (Fontaine et al. 2003).

Drawing on her years of experience as a clinical psychologist, Doreen Samelson provides an excellent guide for what to expect before, during, and after weight loss surgery. Dr. Samelson's book drives home the concept that the long-term success of weight loss surgery is dictated by the collaboration between the patient and her medical team to develop behavioral modifications and lifelong habits that help them reach their goals.

—Arnold D. Salzberg, MD

Introduction

With obvious difficulty, Josie walks into my office and sits down in the oversized chair next to my desk. "I was worried I might have to squeeze into one of those small chairs most doctors have in their offices," she says, shifting her weight in the chair and pulling down her flowered shirt. At age thirty-eight, Josie's obesity is threatening her health and making it increasingly difficult for her to get around. Like many patients I see, Josie is considering weight loss surgery (WLS) and has come to see me for the required presurgery psychological evaluation.

I soon learn that Josie's struggle with weight and weight loss began early. Starting with her first diet at age seven, which was prompted by a trip to her family doctor, Josie recites the long list of diets she has tried. "Losing weight isn't the problem," she explains. "I'm an expert dieter, but each time I lose weight, I gain even more back. The last few years I haven't even bothered to diet." Her discouragement is obvious. However, weight loss surgery isn't for everyone, and I'm not sure Josie is prepared for surgery or ready to accept the consequences of surgically assisted weight loss.

From many years of experience with patients seeking WLS, I know that surgery is never a cure for obesity. Weight regain after surgery, while less common than with conventional dieting, is a real possibility. The excitement people feel the first year after surgery, when pounds come off at an impressive rate, can be replaced by disgust two years after surgery, when the pounds come back and postsurgical food choices feel increasingly constraining.

Josie, a certified public accountant, spends most of her work time at a computer. She explains that she usually skips breakfast and lunch, preferring to snack throughout the afternoon at her desk. A can of diet soda is her constant companion. Josie impresses me with her busy social life, but reveals that most of her friends also struggle with obesity. Their Friday night get-togethers usually consist of trying out a new restaurant. "When I go out to a good restaurant, I sometimes overeat," she admits. Like many of my patients, Josie finds exercise difficult, and she recently received a "handicapped" placard for parking. "I feel a little bad about using it," she says, glancing down at her lap. "I think people are probably looking at me and wondering why I don't just lose weight and leave the handicapped parking spaces to real disabled people."

Despite her comment about "real disabled people," the fact is that Josie's obesity *is* disabling, and it isn't just difficulty walking that interferes with her life. Josie and her doctor are worried about the threat of diabetes. "I know a lot about diabetes, because my mom had it. For the last two years of her life, my mother only left her house when I took her to the doctor. She was sick all the time—it was very depressing. I always knew I could develop diabetes but thought I wouldn't have to think about it until I was older. Now my doctor tells me I have prediabetes." It's clear that Josie's obesity is seriously impacting her health and if something doesn't change, she's at risk of following in her mother's footsteps to an early death.

WEIGHT LOSS SURGERY IS A TOOL

WLS (also called *bariatric surgery*) is not one surgery but a group of surgeries. All commonly performed WLS types decrease the size of your stomach, and some surgeries also change your body's ability to metabolize food, making WLS an effective tool for weight loss. As with all tools, learning to use the WLS tool is essential. If Josie wants WLS, she needs to start making lifestyle changes *before* surgery to prepare for her life after surgery. She needs to learn how to use WLS to lose weight and avoid weight regain. In addition Josie must learn to cope with postsurgery challenges like loose skin and eating restrictions and, more importantly, to change the way she thinks about food and her body.

The increase in frequency of WLS has taught us a lot about what it takes to make this surgery successful. WLS requires that you make permanent lifestyle changes, which means committing yourself to eating an entirely different way for the rest of your life. If you are considering surgery, have decided to have surgery, or already had WLS but are experiencing weight regain, this book can help you successfully lose weight and keep it off. Throughout this workbook you'll be asked to complete WLS activities designed to help you decide whether surgery is your best option, help you prepare for surgery, and help you be successful after surgery.

HOW THIS BOOK IS ORGANIZED

This workbook is divided into three parts:

◆ Part 1, "Making the Decision": WLS is not for everyone, so it's important to explore your reasons for choosing surgery. Chapters 1 through 4 provide you the opportunity to explore the costs and benefits of surgery, learn about the different surgery options, and identify your personal reasons for having WLS. By the end of part 1, you'll know whether WLS is the right choice for you.

◆ Part 2, "Preparing for Success by Taking Action": Preparation is key to achieving sustained weight loss with WLS. Chapters 5 through 12 give you the tools you need to prepare yourself, change your eating habits, and know what to expect when you meet with your surgeon.

◆ Part 3, "Life After Weight Loss Surgery": WLS requires you to make permanent changes in your lifestyle. Chapters 13 through 17 cover preventing weight regain, dealing with loose skin, coping with social situations involving food, and dealing with body-image concerns.

HOW TO USE THIS WORKBOOK

The WLS activities in this workbook are meant to be completed sequentially, starting with chapter 1. If you've already decided to have surgery, you may be tempted to skip part 1. Because the first few chapters help you to identify your personal reasons for having surgery and to understand the negative aspects of WLS, it's best if you resist the urge to forgo part 1. Having a full understanding of the drawbacks and benefits of surgery, and identifying your personal reasons for having surgery, will help you minimize postsurgery problems. Deciding to have WLS is a major decision. If you stay in touch with your personal reasons for undergoing WLS, you can keep yourself motivated to make the lifelong lifestyle changes surgically assisted weight loss requires.

PERSONAL STORIES

As you move through the chapters of this book, in addition to doing WLS activities, you'll meet people, like Josie, who've struggled with obesity. When you read these stories, see if you can relate your struggle with obesity to that of the people in the stories. Let's start by learning a little about the people who will take you through each part of this book:

Josie

We've already met Josie, a thirty-eight-year-old accountant who can't remember ever being thin. A successful professional, Josie would like to start her own accounting business but is afraid her appearance will hold her back. Her employer likes her work, but if she goes out on her own, she'll have to market herself, and Josie is aware that being morbidly obese will affect the way she is perceived in the business world. Unfortunately, Josie's concern is realistic. Studies of weight-based stigmatization indicate that Josie *will* be judged based on her weight (Friedman, Ashmore, and Applegate 2008). Even though she is about two hundred pounds overweight, Josie never considered WLS until her doctor told her she had prediabetes.

Rebecca

Rebecca, a forty-five-year-old married woman, was thin until she gave birth to her first child. Then the pattern of not losing much weight after her first pregnancy was repeated with the birth of her second child. A high-school English teacher with a busy schedule and two teenage sons, Rebecca feels her quality of life is high. Recently diagnosed with hypertension, she is concerned about her health. She hasn't dieted much but did try a low-carbohydrate diet and exercise, which resulted in a forty-pound weight loss. However, she regained the forty pounds when she stopped going to the gym. Though Rebecca's husband thinks she is beautiful at any weight, he's worried about her health. Rebecca is about one hundred pounds overweight.

Mark

Overweight most of his adult life, Mark put on an additional 110 pounds after his divorce eight years ago, bringing his weight to a little over 430 pounds. At age sixty-two and with poorly controlled diabetes, sleep apnea, and arthritis, his obesity severely impacts his ability to live a normal life. After more than thirty years in car sales, Mark has been unable to work for over a year. He needs a knee replacement on both sides, but his orthopedic surgeon says the surgery can't be performed until Mark loses at least 150 pounds. Mark played football in high school and was always a "big guy." When he was younger, he was active for his size and didn't feel that his weight was a disadvantage. Now Mark feels out of breath walking to his car, and going up more than a few stairs has become impossible. While he would like to have a romantic relationship, dating seems out of the question; he believes his obesity is a barrier to meeting women.

Megan

WLS is no longer just for adults, as more adolescents are having the surgery (Zeller et al. 2009). A seventeen-year-old high-school senior, Megan is typical of teens considering WLS. Obese all her life, Megan has a strong family history of obesity. In fact Megan's mother had WLS two years ago. Megan's embarrassment about her weight and her fear of ridicule cause her to decline party invitations. Although the teasing decreased when she got to high school, the memories of the bullying she endured in elementary and junior high school are painful. Megan feels most comfortable around her family, her teachers, and her best friend, who is also obese. An excellent student, Megan has compensated for her obesity by being the "smart girl." Megan puts it this way: "I can hide under the persona of the 'straight-A' student who has the best study notes. If you miss class or didn't do your homework, no problem; just ask the fat girl." With her high GPA and good SAT scores, Megan should have her pick of colleges, but she's afraid to be too far from home, and her parents worry that her fear will hold her back. Megan has not experienced any specific obesity-related health problems yet, but her pediatrician has warned Megan and her parents that she could develop medical problems at a young age if she doesn't lose weight.

IT'S ABOUT QUALITY OF LIFE

As we can see from the stories of Josie, Rebecca, Mark, and Megan, obesity impacts overall quality of life, and there's no area of life it doesn't affect. For people who are obese, quality of life decreases as weight increases (Karlsson et al. 2007). Now take a few moments to consider how obesity has affected you. Complete your first activity: on the following page, write your personal story of obesity, making sure to include how obesity affects you emotionally, how long you've lived with obesity, how your excess weight interferes with your life, and any obesity-related health problems you experience.

WHAT'S NEXT?

WLS can change your life, but it's not for everyone. Now it's time to start the process of deciding whether WLS is the right choice for you. The chapters in part 1 will give you the information you need to understand the costs and benefits of WLS and to examine your personal reasons for choosing the surgery.

My Personal Obesity Story

Part 1

Making the Decision

Though WLS is an effective treatment for extreme obesity, surgery is not the right choice for everyone. Successful long-term weight loss after WLS requires a willingness to make lifestyle changes. We'll start by reviewing the guidelines to qualify for surgically assisted weight loss and then examine surgery costs and benefits. In chapter 2 we'll examine different types of WLS surgery. The type of surgery you get will have implications for how much weight you'll lose and how easy it is to regain it. In chapter 3 we'll explore WLS for those over sixty and under nineteen years of age, as well as discuss special considerations for people whose weight is extremely high. In the last chapter of part 1, you'll have the opportunity to explore your personal reasons for having surgery. WLS alters your digestive system and requires a willingness to live with a digestive system that no longer functions normally. Strong personal reasons for having WLS will help you do what is needed for your new digestive system. By the end of part 1, you'll understand your surgery options and be able to explain how WLS will benefit you, and if you choose WLS, you'll be ready to move on to prepare for the surgery.

Chapter 1

Weight Loss Surgery Costs and Benefits

Josie's experience of regaining more weight than she lost with each diet is the rule, not the exception. While weight regain is possible after WLS, when compared to conventional dieting and exercise, surgery results in greater weight loss and better maintenance of weight loss, and as we'll learn in this chapter, sustained weight loss improves health and quality of life. Still, WLS is not without drawbacks, so it's important to understand the costs of surgery as well as have a realistic understanding of its benefits. Surgery costs aren't limited to insurance co-payments and deductibles. WLS has lifestyle and physical costs as well. The better you understand these costs beforehand, the more successful you'll be. We'll start by examining the qualification guidelines for surgery and then look at how much weight you can expect to lose with WLS.

WHO QUALIFIES FOR WLS?

Most surgical procedures have qualification guidelines, and WLS is no exception. The majority of surgeons and insurance companies in the United States follow the National Institutes of Health (NIH) guidelines. NIH guidelines use *body mass index* (BMI) and obesity-related medical conditions (like diabetes) to determine who qualifies for WLS (Norris 2007). BMI is a body-weight measure that considers your weight and height. Calculate your BMI by taking these steps, or if you prefer, use one of the many online BMI calculators by searching for "body mass index."

BMI Calculation

My weight in pounds: _____

My height in inches: _____

Now put your weight in pounds and height in inches into this formula:

[Your weight in pounds ÷ (Your height in inches x Your height in inches)] x 703

Here's the formula for someone who is 64 inches tall and weighs 250 pounds:

[250 ÷ (64 x 64)] x 703 = 42.9

Based on NIH guidelines, if your BMI is 40 or higher and you have failed multiple times to lose weight with diet and exercise, WLS is probably appropriate for you. If your BMI is 35 to 39, you may still qualify for WLS if you have obesity-related medical conditions like diabetes, hypertension, or sleep apnea that would likely improve with weight loss. In 2010, an FDA panel recommended lowering the minimum BMI guidelines for the LAP-BAND, a popular type of adjustable gastric banding. If the FDA accepts the panel's recommendations, this type of WLS could be available to patients with BMIs as low as 30. Check with your doctor if you are considering WLS and your BMI is lower than 35 (Pollack 2010). It's important to remember that these are just guidelines, and sometimes other factors, such as your personal surgery risks or severity of obesity-related medical conditions, might be more important than your BMI in determining whether WLS is right for you.

REALISTIC EXPECTATIONS

Unrealistic expectations for surgically assisted weight loss are common. Most people think WLS produces bigger weight losses than it actually does (Heinberg, Keating, and Simonelli 2010). Disappointment with weight loss increases your risk for postsurgical problems like depression and weight regain (Kaly et al. 2008). The first step in developing realistic expectations is to calculate your excess weight. Now that you know your BMI, it's time to calculate your excess weight. The amount of excess weight you're carrying is defined as the amount of weight you need to lose to reach the normal BMI range (18.5 to 24.9). Look at the following table to determine how much you need to weigh to have a BMI of 22 (middle of the normal range). The amount of weight you can expect to lose depends, in part, on surgery type, but losing 40 to 70 percent of excess weight is a good WLS outcome (Norris 2007). It's important to remember that we are talking about percent of excess weight, not percent of total weight.

My Realistic Weight-Loss Range

Find your height in inches on this chart. The weight to the right is your weight at a BMI of 22.

BMI of 22					
Height Inches	Pounds	Height Inches	Pounds	Height Inches	Pounds
58	105	65	132	72	163
59	109	66	136	73	166
60	112	67	140	74	171
61	116	68	144	75	176
62	120	69	149	76	180
63	124	70	153	77	185
64	128	71	157	78	190

My current weight: _____

My weight at a BMI of 22: _____

My current weight minus my weight at a BMI of 22: _____ *(my excess weight)*

40 percent of my excess weight: _____

70 percent of my excess weight: _____

The fact that we usually don't see a 100 percent loss of excess weight after WLS means, if you were thin in young adulthood, you probably won't return to being a thin person. The limits on weight loss with WLS also mean, if you're like Josie and have never been thin, you'll probably never be thin.

Last, while it may sound silly to point out that WLS and weight loss won't make you rich or famous, or resolve normal life issues, it's important to make sure you don't expect all your problems to be solved. The good news is that it's realistic to expect WLS to benefit you in some important ways, so let's look at these benefits now.

WLS HEALTH BENEFITS

Excess weight is associated with serious medical conditions. Your doctor may have told you that you need to lose weight for health reasons. Mark's doctor talks to him at every visit about losing weight, and Mark has tried to lose weight. But like Josie, Mark has never been able to lose enough weight to make a significant difference in his health. So losing enough weight and sustaining that weight loss is a WLS benefit for Mark.

Metabolism

It's not just the amount of weight lost or the ability to keep it off that makes WLS beneficial for someone like Mark. WLS can actually speed up your metabolism, which can help resolve metabolism-related conditions like diabetes (Guth and Livingston 2008). *Metabolism* is the process your body uses to convert food into energy. Your *basal metabolic rate* (BMR) dictates how fast your body turns food into energy. If your BMR is high, you convert food into energy or "burn calories" quickly. The faster you convert food into energy, the more calories you can consume without gaining weight. An extremely low BMR means extra pounds will probably accumulate unless you diligently restrict calories.

How high your BMR is set is determined by factors such as age, gender, amount of body fat, and muscle mass. The bad news is that if you're obese, chronic dieting can actually lower your BMR (Kurian, Thompson, and Davidson 2005). The good news is that in addition to reducing your weight, exercise will increase your BMR. Exercise builds muscle, and the higher your muscle mass, the higher your BMR will likely be. Mark is a good example of how muscle mass can make a difference in BMR. Even though Mark was overweight during his football days, he was muscular. His muscular physique, along with his lower weight and age during his teens and twenties, translated into a higher BMR, and Mark found he could eat a lot without gaining weight. In his thirties, Mark maintained his high-school weight but became less active. His change in activity level decreased his muscle mass, adding to the normal age-related decline in his BMR. This decrease in BMR made it easier for Mark to put on weight as he moved into middle age. After his divorce Mark gained more weight, lowering his BMR even more, and he developed serious health problems.

METABOLIC DISEASE

Metabolic disease occurs when your body can't efficiently convert calories into energy. Excess weight around your middle, called *central obesity*, is a risk factor for most metabolic diseases (Nishimura, Manabe, and Nagai 2009). The most common metabolic disease associated with obesity is type 2 diabetes. Type 2 diabetes occurs when your body doesn't recognize insulin (called *insulin resistance*) or doesn't make enough insulin. Without proper amounts of insulin, your body can't metabolize or regulate *glucose*, the major form of sugar in your blood, resulting in high amounts of blood glucose. High blood glucose damages organs and may cause blindness, heart and kidney damage, and sometimes impairs circulation, leading to amputation of toes, feet, and legs. More than 60 percent of the nontraumatic amputations performed in the United States result from diabetes (Dalla Paola and Faglia 2006). Resolution or improvement in type 2 diabetes is one of the major advantages of WLS.

Weight loss has a positive effect on metabolic disease, but WLS can also increase your BMR and improve metabolic disease independent of weight loss. While not all types of WLS confer this metabolic advantage, most types of WLS produce a positive metabolic change. In the next chapter we'll look at which surgeries carry a metabolic advantage.

Life Span

Because obesity is associated with serious health conditions, including some types of cancer, weight loss can increase your life span (Shah, Simha, and Garg 2006). If you're severely obese, WLS will increase your expected life span by about 30 percent (LABS 2009). Resolution of diabetes and decreased risk for some cancers are just two of the reasons for this increase in life span.

Obesity-Related Medical Conditions

WLS can help resolve or improve these medical conditions or physical limitations. Check any conditions you are living with.

- ☐ Type 2 diabetes
- ☐ Hypertension
- ☐ High cholesterol or hyperlipidemia
- ☐ Breathing problems
- ☐ Coronary heart disease
- ☐ Nonalcoholic liver disease
- ☐ Kidney disease
- ☐ Increased cancer risks

- ☐ Gallbladder disease
- ☐ Acid reflux
- ☐ Sleep apnea
- ☐ Polycystic ovary syndrome
- ☐ Chronic back or joint pain, osteoarthritis of the knee
- ☐ Walking limitations
- ☐ Other: _____

WLS AND QUALITY OF LIFE

In addition to improving overall health, weight loss improves overall quality of life, and the more weight an obese person loses, the greater the improvement in quality of life (Karlsson et al. 2007). If you decide to have WLS, you can expect improvement in these areas after weight loss:

◆ Social interactions

- Perception of health, feeling of being healthy

- Self-esteem and body image

- Mood (during the first year)

- Feeling of self-efficacy

Let's look at each of these areas to see how obesity impacts your life and how WLS can improve each area.

Social Interactions

It's not hard to see how obesity affects social interactions. Even though Josie is a social person, her difficulties walking and fitting into an airplane seat or theater seat make it harder for her to enjoy certain social activities. In addition to these physical barriers, obesity affects the way others socially perceive Josie. Social stigmatization of obese people is well documented and affects social interactions with friends, family members, and coworkers. In addition social stigma can lead to job discrimination, making Josie's fear that her obesity will affect her ability to find clients for her future business a realistic concern (Friedman, Ashmore, and Applegate 2008).

It's not just how others treat you; lack of confidence can also be a social roadblock. Megan's lack of social confidence interferes with her social interactions. Having been bullied in the past, Megan is afraid she will be judged for her size, so she stays close to home and avoids social activities. Megan adopted the "smart girl" role as a defense. While it's not a bad role, staying completely within its confines limits her socially.

Not everyone who is obese reports social barriers; some obese people report that their social relationships are not affected significantly by their weight. Remember Rebecca, the high-school teacher? With less weight to lose, a good relationship with her husband, and close relationships with fellow teachers, Rebecca is less socially affected by her weight.

Consider how obesity has affected your social life. Are there social activities you avoid? How are your relationships affected by your weight? In the following space, describe how obesity affects your social interactions.

My obesity affects my social interactions by:

Perception of Health

Perception of health is an important factor in how you feel about yourself. While feeling healthy may or may not correspond to actual physical health, many people who are obese feel unhealthy. Rebecca's extra weight makes her feel unhealthy. And it isn't her hypertension that makes her feel unhealthy, because like most people with hypertension, Rebecca doesn't feel any different when her blood pressure is high. For Rebecca the feeling of being unhealthy is tied to what she sees in the mirror. She puts it this way: "I see the extra weight I've gained and think I look unhealthy even when my blood pressure is controlled." Below, write about how you perceive your health. Do you feel unhealthy because of your weight? If you do feel unhealthy, what is it about being obese that makes you feel unhealthy?

> *My obesity affects my perception of my health by:*

Self-Esteem and Body Image

Self-esteem and body image are related concepts that weight strongly affects. If you're obese, it's hard to have a good self-esteem and body image in a culture that values thinness. The good news is that most people find that their body image and self-esteem improve after WLS.

Self-esteem can be characterized as self-worth or self-pride, but it is sometimes misunderstood as the belief that you can be and do anything. This isn't true for anyone, thin or obese. Similarly, being told how great you are or telling yourself how great you are is not the road to good self-esteem. Much of our feeling of self-worth is derived from our accomplishments. When we accomplish a task, learn something new, or cope with a life challenge, our self-esteem improves. Unfortunately for some obese people, weight overrides accomplishments. For example, despite her intelligence and academic accomplishments, Megan's self-esteem is low. Dismissing her good grades and other assets, Megan describes her self-worth this way: "I'm just the fat girl."

Body image is how you think about or describe your body—what you think you look like. Body image can be distorted. It's not uncommon for an obese person to see herself as more or less obese than she actually is, which is sometimes referred to as having a distorted body image. Rebecca was thin in her teens and early twenties, and kept her thin body image after she gained weight. This is how she explains her distorted body image: "I still see myself as a size 8. I know that's wrong, but when I look in the mirror, I'm surprised to see someone who's a size 22." Distorted body image can also occur in the other direction when formerly obese people are stuck with a "fat" body image. This is a risk for someone like Megan or Josie, who has been obese since childhood. It's possible that both will have to work on changing their body image to match the smaller body that weight loss brings. Because a distorted body image is a common problem, we'll talk more about how to change your body image in part 3. Consider your self-esteem and body image, and describe them in the following space.

My weight affects my self-esteem by:

I see my body as being:

Mood

Most people experience improvements in mood after weight loss surgery. Perhaps because of improved social interactions and self-esteem, as well as better physical health, many people report feeling happier after WLS. However, while we see long-term changes in self-esteem and social interactions, WLS won't cure depression or anxiety in anyone who has chronic or episodically recurrent depression or anxiety. People with a history of psychological disorders like major depressive disorder frequently experience improvements in depression in the year after WLS, but this improvement is often temporary. This is an important point because it appears that symptoms of depression and anxiety are more common in morbidly obese people. Why many people with a history of mood or anxiety disorders return to experiencing depression or anxiety isn't completely understood, but it may be that symptoms rooted in factors less related to weight are less affected by weight loss (Norris 2007). If you have a history of a depressive or anxiety disorder, you don't need to worry that surgery will make your mental health worse, but you may return to your baseline level of depression or anxiety symptoms after WLS (Karlsson et al. 2007). Outside of disorders like major depressive disorder, most people feel happier after losing weight. So it appears that while true psychological disorders aren't cured by weight loss, negative mood associated with the stress of being obese does improve with WLS. In the following space, describe how you think obesity affects your mood.

Obesity interferes with my mood by:

Self-Efficacy

Self-efficacy is your confidence or belief in your ability to take on and successfully deal with life challenges, like employment change or relationship problems. Obesity has a negative effect on self-efficacy, but the good news is that WLS can improve it (Batsis et al. 2009). Megan's reluctance to go away to college could be related to low self-efficacy. She worries about being able to successfully navigate the challenges of living away from her family. Mark feels unable to cope with developing new relationships. He would like to date again and perhaps remarry but feels incapable of negotiating a new relationship. Rebecca, on the other hand, has high self-efficacy. She sees herself as a competent teacher and mother who can deal with her students and teenage sons. Her weight has had little effect on her self-efficacy.

Consider how obesity affects your confidence in coping with life challenges. Do you feel less able to deal with what life brings your way because of your weight? In the following space, write how obesity has affected your confidence.

Being obese affects my confidence in dealing with the challenges of life by:

HEALTH-RELATED QUALITY OF LIFE QUESTIONNAIRE

You've had a chance to consider how being obese affects specific aspects of your quality of life. To see how obesity has affected your overall quality of life, fill out the following questionnaire, using a scale from 1 to 5, where 1 means "strongly disagree" and 5 means "strongly agree."

Obesity-Related Quality of Life Questionnaire

	Rating: 1–5
1. *My obesity has negatively affected my relationships with others.*	
2. *Obesity interferes with my job or career because of social stigma.*	
3. *My obesity prevents me from doing things like going to the movies or taking airline flights because I can't fit into the seats.*	
4. *My weight badly affects my health, and I miss out on doing things I love because of poor health.*	
5. *My self-esteem is very poor.*	
6. *I feel very unattractive.*	
7. *I'm embarrassed by my obesity.*	
8. *Being obese makes me feel emotionally low.*	
9. *I feel incapable of coping with life challenges like looking for a new job.*	
10. *My obesity has had a negative effect on my quality of life.*	
My Total Score	

Score:

40–50	Obesity probably has a strong negative effect on your quality of life.
26–39	Obesity probably has a negative effect on your quality of life.
10–25	Obesity probably has some negative effect on your quality of life.
Below 10	Obesity probably affects your quality of life in minor ways.

THE COST OF LOSING WEIGHT WITH WLS

While it's clear that WLS has lots of benefits, there are also costs of surgery. If you decide to have WLS, you'll go into surgery with a normal digestive system and come out with an abnormal one, and that abnormal gut has far-reaching implications for how you will live your life. The negative side of WLS includes significant restrictions in what you can eat, changes in bowel habits, and problems with vitamin absorption. Because many social interactions involve food or eating, WLS has family-life and social implications. And weight loss itself has some negative aspects. One of the negative aspects is loose skin, which is a common problem when a large amount of weight is lost. Last, WLS sometimes leads to complications like postsurgery infections, and in rare cases people have died due to surgery complications. Let's start by looking at the costs of WLS in terms of how your food choices change after surgery.

Post-WLS Eating

Before WLS you have a wide range of foods to choose from. Even if you're dieting, you might give yourself a small treat as a break from your diet without much negative consequence. After surgery you'll need to limit your food choices permanently. One way to examine this change is to consider a typical dinner. A typical American dinner might include a salad, some kind of meat, and rice or potatoes. Maybe you'd pick an American favorite like fried chicken or, if you're more health conscious, a grilled chicken breast. Most people drink something with dinner, so let's add a glass of wine or soda (diet, of course), and a glass of water. And finally, for dessert, you might have a scoop of ice cream or a piece of fruit and a cup of coffee. This is a pretty basic dinner that draws from the food groups we all learned about in school, right? To see how this typical dinner changes after WLS, let's look at the following chart.

How Dinner Changes After WLS		
Typical Dinner Before WLS	*Dinner After WLS*	*Why*
√ Salad	~~Salad~~	! Your meal should focus on protein, and there's little protein in salad.
√ Rice or potato	~~Rice or potato~~	! Rice expands in the stomach, and potato has little protein (a few small bites of potato is okay).
√ Fried chicken or grilled chicken breast	~~Fried chicken~~	! Fried foods should be avoided and can upset your stomach.
	√ Grilled chicken breast	! Good source of protein; this is the one item on the list you *should* eat.
√ Glass of wine or a diet soda	~~Glass of wine~~ ~~Diet soda~~	! No alcohol after surgery. ! No carbonation of any kind unless you want gas.
√ Glass of water	~~Glass of water~~	! You shouldn't eat and drink at the same time, so even water is out until thirty minutes after your meal.
√ Scoop of ice cream	~~Scoop of ice cream~~	! No sugar; it interferes with weight loss and can make you feel sick.
√ Fruit	~~Fruit~~	! Some fruits are okay, but not ones with lots of fructose (sugar), like pineapple; lower-sugar fruits, like strawberries, are a good choice only in small amounts.
√ After-dinner Coffee	√ After-dinner Coffee	! Decaffeinated coffee is okay (no caffeine), thirty minutes after eating.

Many foods considered part of a normal meal are eliminated after WLS, and protein becomes the main feature of the remaining choices. You should permanently eliminate carbonated or caffeinated drinks from your diet. Carbonation causes gas after surgery, and caffeine is hard on a surgically altered stomach. The metabolism of alcohol is changed after WLS, leading to quick inebriation and possible alcohol dependence. You should eliminate foods like bread and rice, which contain little protein and expand in the stomach. And while it's possible to have small amounts of a low-sugar fruit or vegetable and a very small amount of potatoes or pasta, food choices after surgery translate to protein, protein, and more protein. Eating protein all the time can be boring. A study of people five years after surgery found that most fell off the protein wagon and weren't getting enough protein (Sarwer et al. 2008b). So if you choose WLS and want to be healthy, you'll have to narrow your food options. To see how much you'll have to change what you eat, write what you had for dinner yesterday.

My dinner menu yesterday:

My meal was made up of _____ *% protein.* (100%, 75%, 50%, 25%, less than 25%)

If I were post-WLS, I would have been able to eat _____ *% of my dinner.*
(100%, 75%, 50%, 25%, less than 25%)

Look over your meal and cross out anything you won't be able to eat after WLS. That means crossing out all drinks, fried food, rice or bread, and foods that are high in carbohydrates or sugar. In addition, note how much of your meal was made up of protein and how much of your dinner you would have been able to eat if you were post-WLS.

Bowel Habits and Vitamin Deficiencies

Other costs of surgery include changes in bowel habits and vitamin deficiencies. Diarrhea, loose stools, and constipation are common problems, depending on the type of WLS surgery you have (Potoczna et al. 2008). Eating the wrong foods can make these problems worse, and bowel problems can become chronic.

Vitamin deficiencies are also an important consequence of WLS. While not all types of WLS cause vitamin deficiencies, any WLS that changes your metabolism affects vitamin absorption. Iron, vitamin B_{12}, folate, calcium, and other B-vitamin deficiencies are common (Shah, Simha, and Garg 2006). The change in your body's ability to absorb vitamins after WLS means taking supplements for the rest of your life.

Eating Is a Social Activity

In addition to the postsurgery physical problems like vitamin deficiencies, WLS changes your relationship to social eating. Many social activities involve food. Socializing on Friday nights over dinner at a new restaurant is an important part of Josie's social life. WLS will change her Friday nights. She won't be able to eat many of the foods her friends are enjoying, and she might find eating at a new restaurant each week difficult. Imagine if you went to a new restaurant when you didn't know whether you could eat from its menu. How stressful would that be for you? Would you want to go for the conversation and not eat? Would you take your own food or eat right before going? Or skip the outing? Consider how food is integrated into your social interactions. How often do your social activities involve food? In the following space, list the social activities you engaged in during the last week involving eating or drinking. Be sure to include activities like lunching with coworkers or meeting a friend for coffee.

> *During the last week, I attended these social activities, which included food:*

How many food-related social activities did you engage in? Next write how sticking to the post-WLS eating restrictions will change food-related social activities for you.

> *WLS will change my food-related social activities by:*

Relationships

It's not just sharing a meal in a social setting that changes after WLS; relationships, even friendships, can change after surgery. Megan has one close girlfriend who is also obese. If Megan loses a lot of weight, her weight loss could change her relationship with this friend. The two friends would no longer share the experience of being obese, and it's even possible the friendship wouldn't survive this change. Are most of your friends obese? How do you think losing weight would change your relationships with others?

> *If I lost a lot of weight, it would change my relationships with others by:*

Loose Skin

With lost pounds comes loose skin. Loose skin (also called redundant, excess, or surplus skin) is a cost for the majority of people having WLS (Sarwer et al. 2008a). And this cost can result in actual money out of your pocket if you decide to have loose skin removed. While most insurance companies will pay for surgery to remove loose skin when it's medically necessary (in other words, when the excess skin is causing health problems), excess skin is often not a health problem. Your health insurance won't pay for removal of loose skin that's considered a cosmetic problem. Where the loose skin occurs has important implications for whether your health insurance will cover removal. Removal of loose abdominal skin is sometimes covered by health insurance, while surplus skin hanging off the upper arms, as unsightly as it may be, is rarely considered a health issue and is thus not covered by insurance.

What determines where and how much loose skin you'll experience depends on age, how much weight you lose, where you carry the most weight, and genetics. The younger you are, the less excess skin you'll probably have. The more weight you lose, the more likely you are to have some loose skin. Where you carry the most excess weight is also an important factor in where the loose skin will be. If most of your weight is around your middle, you can expect to have loose abdominal skin. People who carry a lot of excess weight in the upper arms should expect flapping upper arms. It's not uncommon to have more than one area of loose skin. Josie, who has significant central obesity in addition to very large arms and thighs, is at risk for surplus skin in all three areas. Finally your genes play a role in how much loose skin you'll have to contend with. The elasticity of your skin is partly controlled by your genes, and some people just have very elastic skin that tends to snap into a smaller shape with weight loss. If you're lucky enough to have elastic skin, you can thank your parents. Any place you have stretch marks probably won't snap back into place, because stretch marks are an indication that skin has been stretched past its elastic point. To explore your likelihood of having loose skin, answer the following questions.

My Loose Skin Projection

My age is:

- ☐ Under twenty years (1 point)
- ☐ Twenty to thirty years (2 points)
- ☐ Thirty-one to forty years (3 points)
- ☐ Forty-one to fifty years (4 points)
- ☐ Over fifty years (5 points)

I carry a lot of excess weight in my:

- ☐ Abdomen (2 points)
- ☐ Arms (1 point)
- ☐ Neck (1 point)
- ☐ Legs (1 point)
- ☐ Buttocks (1 point)

I have stretch marks in these areas of my body (1 point for each area):

_____

_____

_____

I have family members who've lost weight without much loose skin.   ☐ Yes   ☐ No

(Give yourself 2 points for no and –2 points for yes.)

Total Points: _____

There's no way to know for sure if you'll have loose skin, but in general the higher the points, the more likely you are to have loose skin.

1–3 points: Loose skin is possible.

4–8 points: You'll probably have loose skin on at least one part of your body.

9 points or more: Expect to have significant loose skin on one or more parts of your body.

Surgical Complications

WLS, like all surgeries, carries possible costs in terms of surgical complications. The rate of serious complications and death as a result of WLS is relatively low. The mortality rate for WLS is less than half a percent, with a little over 4 percent of patients experiencing a major complication that requires a longer stay in the hospital or readmission after going home (LABS 2009). The risk of serious complications is greater for people who are older, have multiple health problems, or have a BMI over 60. The good news is that the risks of surgery are balanced by the improved longevity that results from weight loss. While the risks are low and the weight loss WLS brings will probably increase your life span, you should talk to your doctor about your personal risks of surgical complications.

WHAT'S NEXT?

There's more than one type of WLS. It's important to understand the differences, because the type of surgery you have will have implications for how much weight you lose, how easy it will be to regain it, and how much your digestive system is surgically changed. In the next chapter we'll look at the four types of WLS commonly available in the United States as well as the possible medical complications of WLS.

Chapter 2

Not All Weight Loss Surgeries Are Created Equal

In this chapter we'll discuss types of WLS and examine how much each surgery changes the digestive system and the long-term outcome for each surgery. You will decide with your surgeon which surgery to have, and in some cases your health insurance company will be involved in the decision since some companies don't cover all types of WLS. While your preference is a factor, if your chosen option is not medically the best choice for you or your insurance carrier won't approve a certain surgery, you may have to consider another type of WLS. The more you understand the different surgeries, the better prepared you'll be to understand your surgeon's recommendations, ask questions, express your preference, or appeal your insurance company's decision if it denies the WLS your surgeon recommends. Let's start by looking at surgical weight-loss strategies.

STRATEGIES: RESTRICTIVE, MALABSORPTIVE, AND COMBINATION STRATEGIES

WLS strategies either restrict the amount of food you can put in your stomach (*restrictive strategy*) or reduce the calories the small intestine can absorb (*malabsorptive strategy*). The most comprehensive types of WLS use a combination of both strategies. The type of surgery you have has implications for how much weight you lose and how easy it'll be to regain it.

Restrictive Strategy

All forms of WLS commonly available in the United States restrict the usable size of the stomach, resulting in a feeling of fullness after eating a small amount of food. Some surgeries accomplish this by removing part of the stomach, while others section off a part of the stomach so that most of the stomach is unusable.

GASTRIC BANDING

Gastric banding is a group of restrictive-only surgeries. The most popular, *adjustable gastric banding*, involves placing an adjustable band around the top of the stomach to create a small stomach pouch. No part of your stomach is removed, and no changes are made in the small intestine. While gastric banding is not generally meant to be reversible, it *can* be reversed because no part of the stomach is removed. An advantage of gastric banding is that you don't have to worry about taking vitamins, because vitamin absorption isn't affected. While gastric banding changes your digestive system less than other surgeries, its downside is that it's harder to lose weight and keep it off (Tice et al. 2008). Snacking all day or drinking calories can circumvent the effect of having less usable stomach area (Kurian, Thompson, and Davidson 2005). It's also possible to expand the size of the stomach pouch or cause the band to slip by overeating (Bueter et al. 2008).

You can expect to lose up to 40 to 50 percent of your excess weight with a gastric band, but the risk of weight regain is high. Five years after surgery, 25 to 33 percent of gastric banding recipients regain most or all lost weight. As a result, the rate of *revisional*, or second, surgeries due to inadequate weight loss is higher for gastric banding than for other surgeries (Strain et al. 2009).

GASTRIC SLEEVE

First developed for patients needing to lose weight prior to combination surgery, the *gastric sleeve* (also called *sleeve gastrectomy*) is a newer surgery that's now done as a stand-alone surgery. This is a restrictive surgery that makes a sleeve or small tube out of the stomach by removing much of your stomach. Unlike gastric banding, the change in stomach size is irreversible, and there's no band to adjust or slip, but you can stretch out the stomach sleeve if you overeat. Though there's less research on the gastric sleeve, the early results suggest weight loss is better one year after surgery than with gastric banding. Resolution of diabetes may be as good as with surgeries using a malabsorptive strategy. Long-term outcome with the gastric sleeve isn't known; it may be that, as with gastric banding, it's easier to regain weight (Lakdawala et al. 2010).

Malabsorptive Strategy

In a normal digestive system, the upper part of the small intestine, attached to the stomach, absorbs a large portion of the calories we consume. *Malabsorption* is achieved by bypassing, but not removing, this upper part of the small intestine so that food no longer passes though this part of your digestive system, resulting in fewer calories being absorbed and improved metabolism. Because vitamins are also normally absorbed in the upper part of the intestine, vitamin absorption is affected. In addition to problems with vitamin absorption, bypassing the upper part of the small intestine can lead to something called *sugar dumping*. While not everyone who has surgery employing malabsorption experiences sugar dumping, if you do experience sugar dumping, you'll feel very sick after eating or drinking something with a high sugar or fat content (for more about sugar dumping, see the text box in this chapter, "Sugar Dumping: Friend or Foe?"). In the United States, surgeries that employ the malabsorptive strategy always combine malabsorption with restriction. So when you talk with a WLS surgeon, you'll be discussing either restrictive surgery or a combination surgery that uses both strategies.

Combination Surgeries

Combined surgeries take advantage of both WLS strategies. Combination surgeries lead to greater weight loss and are associated with less weight regain. The most common WLS performed in the United States is a combination surgery called the *Roux-en-Y gastric bypass*.

ROUX-EN-Y GASTRIC BYPASS

The Roux-en-Y gastric bypass (often shortened to RNYGB) accounts for about 80 percent of all WLS performed in the United States (Adams et al. 2007). When performing the RNYGB, the surgeon makes a small stomach pouch that can hold about two ounces of food, bypasses the upper part of the small intestine, and removes the strong ring of muscles connecting the stomach to the intestine. Called the *pyloric valve*, this ring of muscles controls how quickly food is moved into the small intestine. The removal of the pyloric valve causes food to move more quickly into the intestine. The RNYGB has many advantages. Compared to gastric banding, the RNYGB leads to better weight loss, less weight regain, and more-frequent improvement or resolution of obesity-related conditions like diabetes (Tice et al. 2008). The RNYGB requires that you take vitamins for the rest of your life, and the lack of a pyloric valve means you may experience sugar dumping.

THE DUODENAL SWITCH

Also called *biliopancreatic diversion with duodenal switch* or *gastric reduction duodenal switch*, the *duodenal switch* surgically decreases the size of the stomach using the gastric sleeve method, and bypasses part of the small intestine. But unlike in the RNYGB, the pyloric valve isn't removed. Preserving the pyloric valve decreases the chances of sugar dumping. While some studies show greater weight loss compared to the RNYGB (Topart, Becouarn, and Ritz 2007), recent studies found more extreme vitamin deficiencies with the duodenal switch (Aasheim et al. 2009). Because the expected weight loss difference between the duodenal switch and RNYGB isn't great and the nutrient problems after duodenal switch are greater, some surgeons prefer the RNYGB (Strain et al. 2009).

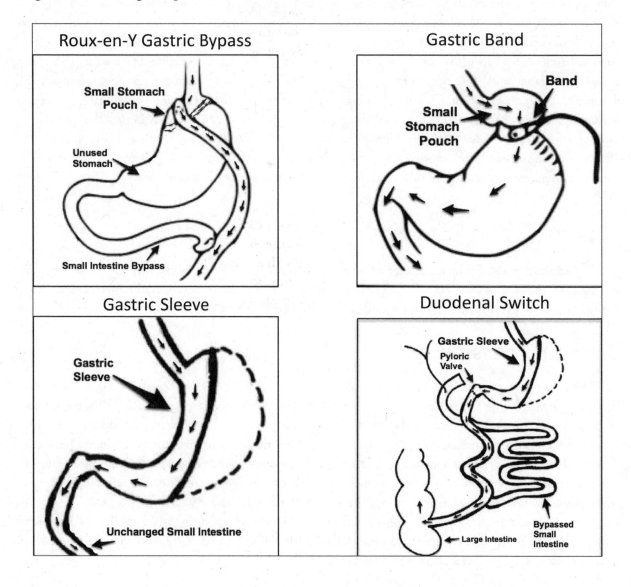

Sugar Dumping: Friend or Foe?

Also called rapid gastric emptying, sugar dumping occurs most often with RNYGB. Dumping occurs because food, which under normal circumstances sits in the stomach before moving in a controlled manner into the small intestine, no longer takes that normal course. Without the pyloric valve, food is quickly "dumped" into the intestine. Sugar dumping occurs with high-sugar foods (even some fruits) or high-fat foods. Symptoms include:

◆ Nausea

◆ Vomiting

◆ Sweating

◆ Abdominal pain and cramps

◆ Diarrhea

◆ Dizziness

◆ Bloating and belching

◆ Fatigue

◆ Heart palpitations

The bad news about sugar dumping is also the good news. The miserable symptoms can keep you on the right path. As you can probably imagine, the threat of experiencing these symptoms will make you think twice about eating something with a lot of sugar or fat. Not everyone who has RNYGB experiences sugar dumping, and over time the frequency and severity of dumping can lessen or disappear, making it gradually easier to eat the wrong foods (Kurian, Thompson, and Davidson 2005).

MEDICAL RISKS

While most people who have WLS experience few or no medical complications, in the excitement of potential weight loss, it's easy to forget that, as with all surgeries, serious medical complications are possible (Madan, Tichansky, and Taddeucci 2007). These complications can be divided into early and late complications. Early complications are problems that occur around the time of surgery, and they range from death to wound infections. Death is rare but can occur with WLS. Late complications are problems that occur after recovery from surgery, and they include nutrient deficiencies and band slippage. Factors such as age, BMI, and your overall health are important in determining the risk of complications (Berarducci 2007). In chapter 11 we'll explore what questions to ask your surgeon. For now read through the list of possible WLS complications and circle any that you want to learn more about.

Possible Medical Complications of WLS		
Surgical Strategy	*Early*	*Late*
Restrictive Surgery	Infection Injury to the stomach Band leaks Breathing or lung problems Blood clots Hemorrhage Death	Band slipping or leaking Band erosion Repeated band adjustments Stomach pouch expansion Stomach upset, reflux Weight regain Inadequate weight loss
Malabsorption and Combination Surgery	Infection Hemorrhage Injury to digestive system Breathing or lung problems Bowel obstructions Death	Hernias Diarrhea, gas, bloating, constipation Bowel obstruction Blockage at junction between stomach and intestine Malnutrition Ulcer Weight regain Inadequate weight loss

METHODS: OPEN VS. LAPAROSCOPIC SURGERY

Two surgical methods are used to perform WLS surgery: the *open method* and the *laparoscopic method*. The open surgical method involves one large incision. In contrast, during laparoscopic surgery, the surgeon makes several small incisions. Specialized tools, including a tube attached to a camera small enough to be inserted through the other small incisions are used to perform the surgery. In recent years a dramatic decrease in the number of open surgeries has occurred, and laparoscopic surgery has become the norm (Hinojosa et al. 2009). The advantages of laparoscopic surgery include less recovery time and less postoperative pain. There's no difference in the amount of weight lost or the risk of weight regain between the two surgery methods. While most WLS is now done laparoscopically, open WLS is still performed. Occasionally a surgery starts out as a laparoscopic surgery but becomes an open surgery because the surgeon has to make a large incision to deal with scar tissue or bleeding. This isn't a common occurrence, but if it happened, you could wake up from surgery finding that you had open, rather than laparoscopic, surgery (Kurian, Thompson, and Davidson 2005).

WHAT'S NEXT?

WLS is a useful tool for people of all ages and for those with extremely high BMIs. In the next chapter we'll explore WLS for youths and for people over sixty years old, as well as look at the special considerations for people with BMIs over 60.

Chapter 3

Weight Loss Surgery for Special Groups

Ten years ago a discussion of special consideration for adolescents aged twelve to nineteen, adults over age sixty, and people who are *superobese* (with a BMI over 60) would have been unnecessary, because people in these three groups rarely had WLS. Now WLS is an option if you fall into one of these groups. We'll start our discussion with youths and WLS.

YOUTHS

Obesity in adolescence has implications for physical and psychological health during adulthood. Compared to obese adults who weren't obese as children, adults with a history of obesity in childhood or adolescence are more likely to develop health problems, to die from those conditions, and to experience depression (Pratt et al. 2009). These sobering facts mean that addressing obesity in a young person like Megan has far-reaching implications.

The first adolescent bariatric surgeries were performed in the 1970s, but the number of surgeries performed was limited. Currently RNYGB and gastric banding are the most common types of bariatric surgery done in adolescents (O'Brien et al. 2010). Because WLS in youth has lagged behind other WLS, we have fewer long-term studies to guide us. What we do know is that young people may not lose as much weight as adults. It can be difficult for anyone, regardless of age, to stick to the postsurgery food rules, but teens may have more difficulties than adults doing so (Xanthakos 2008). In addition it appears that adolescents may be at greater risk for developing eating disorders and depression after WLS, making it imperative that families watch for these problems and give young people access to support from a mental health provider if they occur (Kim et al. 2008).

RNYGB

Despite concerns about WLS for youths, there's a lot of good news. Megan and other teens can expect RNYGB to improve health and quality of life. Similar to adults, youths see improvements in health problems like type 2 diabetes, nonalcoholic fatty liver, and sleep apnea (Pratt et al. 2009). In addition, six to twelve months after surgery, adolescents report:

◆ Improvements in physical abilities like bending over

◆ Less body shame

◆ Higher self-esteem

◆ Less ridicule from peers

Interestingly these improvements occur even when a teen loses only a small of amount of weight (Zeller et al. 2009).

Gastric Banding

One of the few studies to look at gastric banding in youths found that compared to conventional diets, gastric banding resulted in greater weight loss (O'Brien et al. 2010). While these results are promising, concern has been raised about placing a banding device in a young person, who is expected to live with the device much longer than an adult would (Xanthakos 2008). Long-term studies in adolescents with gastric banding will be needed before we'll know if obese teens like Megan can maintain weight loss with the gastric band or will develop problems with the band over time.

Special Word for Parents and Guardians

It's hard for a parent to watch a child struggle with obesity and the problems it brings. Surgery can seem like the solution to your child's struggle, but it's important for you, as a parent or guardian, to consider whether this is the right time for your adolescent to have WLS. Consider how WLS might affect your developing child while he is also experiencing the rapid physical and emotional changes adolescence brings (Zeller et al. 2009). Adolescents don't think like adults because their brains haven't fully matured yet, and the maturity level of individual teens can differ greatly; some sixteen-year-olds are very mature, while others are more childlike. If your young person has never been able to stick to a diet for even a short time, he may lack the maturity and understanding to adhere to the post-WLS lifestyle. Families with frequent parent–teen conflict may find that the young person rejects the support needed to prepare for surgery and to adhere to the postsurgery food rules. In these situations, helping your young person with a conventional diet and exercise program until he has developed the maturity WLS requires may be the best choice.

Discussing the Options

We've learned that there's good news about youths and surgery but also some cause for concern. If you're a teen or the parent of a teen, it's important to talk about the special issues WLS poses for a young person. Taking the time to answer these questions is a good way to start this discussion. You can sit down together to answer them, or answer them separately and discuss your answers—just don't skip the discussion.

Questions for Youth	*Questions for Parents and Guardians*
1. When you tried to lose weight, what was the hardest part about sticking to a diet?	1. How long has your teen been able to stick to a diet program?
2. How long did you stick to the diet?	2. How much support did your teen need from you to stick to a diet?
3. After WLS you will have to eat very differently than your friends do. How will you handle that?	3. How will you support your teen during surgery preparation?
4. How would you like your family to support you in staying on track with eating after WLS?	4. How do you plan to support your teen after WLS?
5. What scares you the most about WLS?	5. If your teen has surgery, what worries you the most?
6. Do you do any binge eating? If you binge eat, do you know what triggers binge eating?	6. Does your teen binge eat? If he does, how will you help him control his eating?
7. Have you been troubled by depression? If you have experienced depression, are you open to getting help for it?	7. Has your teen experienced depression? If so, how are you prepared to help him if he becomes depressed after WLS?
8. Do you know anyone who has had WLS who can support you?	8. Do you know someone who has had WLS who can mentor your teen?
9. Do you plan to live with your parents for at least one year after surgery? If not, will you be living in an environment that will support you in your weight loss?	9. Will your teen be living with you for at least one year after surgery? If not, how will your teen get support after WLS?

How did your discussion go? What conclusions did you come to? When Megan and her parents sat down to talk, they came to these conclusions:

1. Megan was able to stick to a diet for three months, mostly on her own, with help from a dietitian and encouragement from her parents.

2. Megan's mother had WLS and is doing well postsurgery. The family has already made changes in the way they shop and cook, which could help Megan.

3. Megan's best friend is supportive but knows little about WLS. Megan's extended family members are very supportive, and there's a high degree of knowledge about WLS in the family.

4. Megan has a good understanding of the postsurgery lifestyle from watching her mother, who adheres strictly to postsurgery rules.

5. Megan occasionally binges on candy, usually when she feels stressed about school.

6. Megan's parents worry that she might not lose as much weight as she expects. They're afraid this disappointment could lead to weight regain or depression.

7. Megan has experienced some mild depression in the past. She's willing to talk to her school counselor again or go to the college counseling center if she feels depressed after surgery.

As we can see from this summary, Megan and her family have started to address important issues around WLS. On the following page, write a summary of your family discussion.

Summary of my WLS family discussion:

Consider your family's discussion as a starting point. It's important to continue the dialogue as you learn more about WLS. If, after several discussions, you're still not sure this is the best time for WLS, consider starting with conventional diet and exercise.

THE OVER-SIXTY CROWD

At sixty-two, Mark, the man you read about earlier in this book, will need to consider his age in deciding on WLS. Every birthday you celebrate after sixty increases your surgical risks. Older adults have also often lived with obesity-related health conditions like type 2 diabetes for a longer time, which means that someone over sixty may be less healthy going into surgery. Let's look at the increased risks for older adults like Mark (Gómez, Riall, and Gómez 2008):

- *Death:* The risk of dying from surgical complications during or shortly after any kind of surgery is higher for older adults.

- *Surgical complications:* Older adults are at greater risk for surgical complications.

- *Longer hospital stays:* Older adults may need more time to recover from surgery.

- *Rehospitalization:* Like those occurring early after surgery, late complications occur more often in older adults, sometimes requiring rehospitalization.

Despite these concerns, WLS can be safely performed on people over sixty. WLS extends life span in older adults by improving or resolving obesity-related health problems, and improvements in health exceed those seen with conventional dieting. Like in younger adults, amount of weight loss depends on type of surgery, and older adults lose about the same amount of excess weight as younger adults having the same surgery (Wittgrove and Martinez 2009). So if you're over sixty, you and your doctor will need to balance the risks of not having WLS with the risks of having it.

SUPEROBESITY

A BMI of 60 or above (sometimes called *superobesity*) affects WLS outcome. If your BMI is 60 or above, compared to someone with a BMI under 60 (LABS 2009):

- Your risk of dying from obesity-related health conditions is higher.

- Your risk of death or serious complications with any kind of surgery is higher.

- You may need an open WLS.

- You'll likely lose less weight with WLS than people with a lower BMI. For this reason, some experts don't recommend gastric banding for someone with an extremely high BMI.

- You'll probably have significant amounts of loose skin after weight loss.

WHAT'S NEXT?

Thus far we have explored what WLS can do for you, how WLS surgeries differ, and how living after WLS compares to living with a normal digestive system, plus we've looked at special considerations for youths, people over sixty, and those with an extremely high BMI. Now it's time for you to decide whether WLS is the best weight-loss tool for you.

Chapter 4

Is Weight Loss Surgery the Right Tool for You?

In this chapter you'll determine whether WLS is the best weight-loss tool for you. Because it helps to consider your diet and weight-loss history in making the decision, we'll start with a personal diet and weight-loss history. By now you are aware that WLS permanently changes your digestive system. We'll look at what it means to be willing to accept the new digestive-system changes WLS produces. If this isn't your first WLS, you'll look at what you need to do differently this time around. Finally you'll explore your personal compelling weight-loss goal and complete a WLS cost-benefit analysis, which will help you arrive at a decision.

PERSONAL DIET AND WEIGHT-LOSS HISTORY

Even if you've dieted only once or twice, you probably managed to stay on a diet for a short time and lost a few pounds. Three good reasons to examine your diet and weight-loss history are: First, figuring out what strategies have worked for you in the past can help you lose weight and sustain that weight loss with conventional dieting if you decide surgery isn't the right tool for you. Second, you can expect to be asked about your history of dieting and weight loss as part of your pre-WLS medical and psychological evaluations. Last, some health insurance companies require a history of failed dieting before they will approve WLS, so you may have to document this information on insurance forms.

Weight Loss Strategies

WLS means changing how you eat for the rest of your life. The good news is if you choose WLS, dieting has probably taught you some strategies that will help you adhere to the restrictive postsurgery lifestyle. Weight loss strategies abound. Look at these common dieting strategies and check those you've tried:

- ☐ Increasing physical activity
- ☐ Ridding your home of unhealthy foods
- ☐ Meal planning
- ☐ Writing down in a log everything you eat
- ☐ Weighing yourself regularly (at least once a week)
- ☐ Eating out less often
- ☐ Eating prepackaged diet food
- ☐ Using liquid meal replacements
- ☐ Joining a weight-loss group for support or coaching
- ☐ Other: _____

Which strategies resulted in the most weight loss? What helped you keep weight off, even if it was for only a few months?

The weight loss strategies that helped me lose weight were:

The strategies that helped me keep weight off for even a few months were:

When Rebecca completes these sentences, she realizes that dieting without exercise is a mistake. It isn't just burning calories that helps her; she feels healthier when she goes to the gym, so she eats healthier. When completing these sentences, Mark recalls that what he keeps in his kitchen makes a difference. As he puts it, "If I have ice cream or chips in the house, the diet goes out the window." Since eating ice cream or chips after WLS could sabotage Mark's weight loss, keeping these foods out of his house will help him stay on track after WLS. Megan has dieted only once, after consulting with a dietitian who helped her with a meal plan. Meal planning is a tool Megan can use.

Compiling Your Diet and Weight-Loss History

In addition to completing the information on weight loss strategies, it's a good idea to think about when you first dieted and note the formal diets you have tried. Fill out this questionnaire with your diet and weight-loss history. You'll probably be asked these questions in at least one of your presurgery medical appointments.

My Diet and Weight-Loss History Questionnaire

1. *I started dieting at age* _____ .

2. *I've stayed on a diet for at least one week* _____ *times in my life.*

3. *The most I ever lost while dieting was* _____ *pounds.*

4. *The longest I kept off ten pounds or more was* _____ *weeks/months (circle one).*

5. *I've tried over-the-counter diet pills.* ☐ Yes ☐ No

6. *I've tried prescription diet pills.* ☐ Yes ☐ No

7. *I've tried these diets (if you're a chronic dieter, list your last five diets):*

   _____

   _____

   _____

8. *Most of the time I regained more than I lost.* ☐ Yes ☐ No

---

WILLINGNESS

WLS requires *willingness*. Willingness means accepting what's true about you and your body and doing what's effective for your body and life. Willingness isn't the same as wanting something. Most people who are obese want to be thinner. But if just wanting to be thin made people thin, this book would be unnecessary. After WLS, willingness is accepting that your digestive system will be permanently changed and that you'll have to eat differently than someone with a normal digestive system does. Unlike dieting, WLS means permanent changes in how and what you eat.

Trying to eat the way you did before surgery is a refusal to be willing, which leads to poor weight loss and to problems like sugar dumping and weight regain. We call this refusal *willfulness*. Willfulness is the opposite of willingness. An example of being willful is eating bread, which has little protein and can expand the size of your stomach. The more willful you are after surgery, the less weight you'll lose and the more likely you'll regain weight. By now you have a good idea of how you'll have to eat after WLS. Consider all you've learned about postsurgery eating, and answer this willingness question:

Am I willing to accept a surgically altered digestive system that will affect how and what I eat for the rest of my life?   ☐ Yes   ☐ No   ☐ Not sure

---

If you answered yes to this question, you're willing to make the changes WLS requires for successful weight loss and maintenance. If you answered no or "not sure," you have some thinking to do. It doesn't really matter what your reasons are for losing weight or how much you want to lose weight; if you can't accept a changed digestive system that necessitates eating differently, surgery isn't the right weight-loss tool for you. If you find yourself in this situation, take some time to:

◆ Think about what you have learned so far about WLS.

◆ Make a list of foods you think you might have difficulty giving up. Look over the list and ask yourself how important these foods are. Could you consider permanently giving up these foods if it meant better health?

◆ Talk to your friends and family. How supportive of your having WLS are the people close to you?

◆ Find someone who has had WLS to find out firsthand how hard it is to eat after surgery.

◆ Take your time; don't rush. Consider moving on to the next section of the book while keeping in mind that having surgery before you're willing will sabotage your success.

REVISIONAL SURGERIES: WHEN IT'S NOT YOUR FIRST WEIGHT LOSS SURGERY

Sometimes one WLS is not enough, so a revisional (second) WLS is needed. The most common reasons for revisional WLS are inadequate weight loss, weight regain, and intractable surgical complications. Inadequate weight loss and weight regain are, by far, the most frequent reasons for a revision. If we look at revisions done for inadequate weight loss or weight regain, gastric banding has the highest revision rate (Marsk et al. 2009). Revision from gastric banding to combination surgery has the highest second-surgery success rate. However, if your first WLS was a combination surgery, adding a gastric band for additional stomach restriction can improve weight loss (Brolin and Cody 2008).

If you're considering a second WLS because of inadequate weight loss or weight regain, you must be willing to look at what you did after your first surgery that might have led to poor results, and commit yourself to making different choices the second time around. Answer the following questions about your first WLS surgery.

Inadequate Weight Loss and Weight Regain Questionnaire

1. Did you follow postsurgery eating guidelines? ☐ Yes ☐ No

   If not, why not? _____

   _____

   What has changed that would allow you to follow postsurgery guidelines now?

   _____

2. Did you have good support from family or friends? ☐ Yes ☐ No

   If not, what can you do to get good support now? _____

   _____

   _____

3. Did you avoid snacking? ☐ Yes ☐ No

   If you snacked, how can you avoid snacking this time? _____

   _____

4. Did you eliminate emotional or binge eating? ☐ Yes ☐ No

   If not, what is your plan now to eliminate emotional or binge eating? _____

   _____

5. Did you avoid drinking high-calorie drinks? ☐ Yes ☐ No

   If not, what's your plan to eliminate drinking extra calories now?

   _____

6. Did you eliminate foods like bread that expand in the stomach? ☐ Yes ☐ No

   If not, what's your plan to stop eating these foods? _____

   _____

7. Were you exercising at least three to four times a week? ☐ Yes ☐ No

If not, what's your plan to start an exercise program? _____

_____

8. Did you miss any of your follow-up appointments? ☐ Yes ☐ No

If you missed appointments in the past, how will you make sure to go to your follow-up appointments this time? _____

_____

_____

How many no answers do you have? Every no answer is a possible reason for your disappointing results. Don't move ahead with a second WLS unless you really believe you can turn every no answer into a yes this time around.

Check the help or tools you plan to employ for your revision:

☐ Consult a dietitian.

☐ Seek treatment for emotional or binge eating.

☐ Attend a post-WLS support group.

☐ Make a commitment to regular exercise.

☐ Talk to my family and friends about what you need from them to make your revision work.

As you work through the rest of the book, you'll find lots of information that can make your revisional WLS a success, but you must be willing to use that information. If you're still engaging in emotional or binge eating, it's a good idea to see an eating disorder specialist before having a second surgery. If you don't resolve these problems, you may find that your second surgery isn't any more successful than your first. Finally, don't let yourself get discouraged; sometimes all it takes to be successful is a little practice and the opportunity to learn from experience.

PERSONAL COMPELLING GOAL FOR LOSING WEIGHT

A compelling goal is something you're willing to make sacrifices for. A compelling goal can help you keep yourself motivated to do what is needed to make your WLS a success. Your compelling goal must be so important that:

♦ It helps you stay willing and fend off willfulness.

♦ You're willing to have a surgeon change your digestive system in order to achieve sustained weight loss.

Rather than develop a compelling goal that states how much weight you want to lose, consider what you want to accomplish by losing weight. For example, Josie's compelling goal is to resolve her prediabetes, which she believes could cut her life short. Rebecca has a similar compelling goal: to control her high blood pressure. Mark wants to lose enough weight to have his knee replaced and return to his work as a car salesman. Megan's compelling goal is to feel more confident and improve her self-esteem. Next, write your compelling goal:

My compelling goal is:

Can You Accomplish Your Goal Without WLS?

Now that you've identified your compelling goal, it's time to ask yourself if you can accomplish your goal without WLS. When Josie and Rebecca ask themselves this question, they come up with different answers. Josie's BMI is very high. She has little confidence in her ability to keep weight off with conventional dieting, and an examination of her diet and weight-loss history reveals many failed diets. In addition to weight loss, the metabolic advantage of a combination surgery will help Josie resolve her prediabetes. For both of these reasons, she feels fairly sure that she won't be successful in accomplishing her goal without WLS. In contrast, Rebecca's goal of controlling her high blood pressure might be accomplished without surgery. Rebecca has only dieted once and lost forty pounds, which she kept off until she stopped exercising. After talking with her doctor, Rebecca estimates that a thirty-pound weight loss will probably be enough to control her high blood pressure and she can lose this amount of weight without WLS.

Do you think you can reach your compelling goal without WLS? Answer the following questions to see if you can.

> *My compelling goal is:* _____
>
> *I think I would have to lose about* _____ *pounds to reach my compelling goal.*
>
> *Based on my weight-loss and diet history, it's:*
>
> ☐ Realistic that I could lose this much weight without WLS
>
> ☐ Unrealistic to think I could lose this much weight without WLS

Is There a Reason Not to Have WLS?

The last step before moving on to your Personal WLS Cost-Benefit Analysis is to ask yourself if there are any reasons not to have WLS. Reasons for rejecting WLS as a weight-loss tool range from fear of surgery complications to lack of family support. When Rebecca asks herself this question, in addition to the possibility that she might be able to lose enough weight to control her high blood pressure with conventional diet and exercise, a discussion with her husband reveals that he would prefer that Rebecca not have WLS. However, he's very willing to support her in a diet and exercise plan, and he even offers to join her at the gym four times a week, which Rebecca knows will help keep her on track with exercise. When considering this question, Megan and her family wonder if the timing is right. Going off to college is a big change for a young person, and Megan and her mother question whether it's a good idea to transition to both college and the post-WLS lifestyle at the same time. Is there a reason you might not choose WLS?

My Personal Reasons for Not Having WLS

☐ I think I might be able to lose weight without surgery.

☐ I'm afraid of the potential complications of surgery.

☐ My family would prefer that I not have surgery.

☐ I am experiencing so much change in my life right now that it's not a good time to have surgery.

☐ I'm not sure I'm willing to change the way I eat enough to follow postsurgery food rules.

☐ Other: _____

☐ I can't think of a reason not to have WLS.

PERSONAL COST-BENEFIT ANALYSIS

Reflecting on what you have learned about WLS and your own motivations, it's time to fill out your personal cost-benefit analysis. In your cost-benefit analysis, you'll compare what you want to achieve as a result of WLS with what WLS would require you to do or cost you in terms of lifestyle. You'll start by examining your personal benefits. In the "Personal WLS Benefits" column, consider each possible benefit and write why it's important to you:

Personal WLS Cost-Benefit Analysis	
Personal WLS Benefits	*Why This Is Important to Me*
Losing and sustaining at least 40 to 70 percent loss of excess weight	_____ _____ *To be a real benefit to me, the amount of weight I need to lose is at least:* ☐ 40 percent of my excess weight ☐ 50 percent of my excess weight ☐ 60 percent of my excess weight ☐ 70 percent of my excess weight
Being able to fit into an airplane seat or theater seat	_____ _____ ☐ Not important or doesn't apply to me
Improving chronic medical conditions (such as diabetes)	_____ _____ ☐ Not important or doesn't apply me
Improved ability to walk and get around	_____ _____ ☐ Not important or doesn't apply to me

Improved self-esteem	_____ _____ ☐ Not important or doesn't apply to me
Improved body image; feeling more attractive	_____ _____ ☐ Not important or doesn't apply to me
Feeling more confident in dealing with life's challenges	_____ _____ ☐ Not important or doesn't apply to me
Being more energetic and physically active	_____ _____ ☐ Not important or doesn't apply to me
Other benefits:	_____ _____

Now that you've looked at your potential benefits, it's time to examine your personal costs of having WLS. Remember, by costs we're not talking about financial costs, although you certainly should check with your health insurance carrier to see what WLS financial costs are covered. The costs to focus on in deciding whether WLS is the right tool for you are lifestyle costs. For each cost, describe how you will deal with the cost. For example, will you change the way you eat by keeping certain foods out of the house and planning your meals ahead of time? Or maybe you'll write down how much protein you have at each meal to make sure you're getting enough. Costs require willingness to change, so for each cost, rate your willingness on a scale from 0 to 5, with 0 meaning "not willing to pay the price" and 5 meaning "extremely willing."

My Personal Costs

Personal WLS Costs	How I Will Deal with This Cost
Changing the way I eat (focusing on protein and giving up bread, rice, and other foods that aren't healthy after WLS)	Willingness Rating: _____
Giving up alcohol and caffeine for the rest of my life	Willingness Rating: _____
Dealing with interference in my social activities (such as being unable to eat a normal restaurant meal with friends)	Willingness Rating: _____
Having to take vitamin supplements for the rest of my life	Willingness Rating: _____
Dealing with changes in bowel habits (constipation or loose stool)	Willingness Rating: _____
Coping with loose skin	Willingness Rating: _____
Taking time off work for the surgery	Willingness Rating: _____
Having a surgically altered digestive system	Willingness Rating: _____
Dealing with surgical complications	Willingness Rating: _____
Dealing with monetary costs (such as co-pays or deductibles)	Willingness Rating: _____
Other costs: _____	Willingness Rating: _____

Your Decision

Now that you have examined your compelling goal, your personal benefits of WLS, your personal costs, and your willingness to pay those costs, it's time to decide whether WLS is the right tool for you. After carefully looking at her costs and benefits, her level of willingness, and her reasons not to have WLS, Rebecca decides to give herself one year to get her high blood pressure under control with conventional dieting and exercise. After talking with her doctor, Rebecca believes she can reach her compelling goal of blood pressure control with a thirty-pound weight loss. Along with the possibility that she could control her blood pressure with a thirty-pound weight loss, Rebecca decides she isn't willing to accept a surgically changed digestive system and feels the changes she would have to make in her lifestyle would interfere with her life too much. Last, Rebecca considers her husband's preference. She knows that if she had WLS, his support would be important, and she doesn't want to put him in the situation of supporting WLS when he has reservations. Mark and Josie decide to move forward with WLS. The many failed diets and the amount of weight both need to lose to improve their health lead them to decide that WLS is the right tool. After a lot of thought and conversation, Megan and her family still aren't sure Megan is ready for WLS. Sometimes it takes extra time to make this important decision. With her family's support, Megan decides to move ahead and prepare for WLS while continuing to consider her options. The good news is preparation for surgery can improve health and often leads to a small amount of weight loss, so it makes sense for Megan to move ahead with preparation. Next, check your decision:

☐ I have a compelling goal that WLS can help me attain. The benefits of WLS outweigh the costs for me. I am willing to do what it takes to make WLS the right tool for me.

☐ I'm not sure whether the benefits of WLS outweigh the costs. I might be able to achieve my compelling goal without surgery, but I'm not sure. I'll move on to WLS preparation while continuing to consider WLS and how willing I am to make the changes surgery requires.

☐ I think WLS may be the tool I need to reach my compelling goal, but this isn't the right time for me to have surgery. I'll work on improving my health, and I'll consider WLS when the timing is better.

☐ The costs of WLS outweigh the benefits for me, and at this point in my life, I am not willing to make the kinds of changes I would need to make to ensure success after surgery. I'll work on achieving my compelling goal with conventional diet and exercise.

If you decided that surgery is the right tool for you or if you need more time to decide, move on to part 2 and learn how to prepare for WLS. If you think WLS is the right tool but the timing is wrong, you can still benefit from reading chapters 5 through 9. By following the information on eating and exercising in these chapters, you can improve your health while waiting for a better time to consider surgery. Similarly if you are like Rebecca and think you can reach your compelling goal without surgery, you may still want to move on to part 2. Much of the information and most of the activities in chapters 5 through 9 will help you with conventional diet and exercise. If you've decided against surgically assisted weight loss, look for this symbol ❈ in chapters 5 through 9, which will alert you that the information in that section is relevant to both conventional dieting and WLS.

WHAT'S NEXT?

Without adequate preparation for WLS, you'll be at risk for inadequate weight loss and regain. Preparation means taking action, and action requires a willingness to change. In each chapter in part 2, starting with an exercise plan, you'll be asked to take action. Each action will move you toward WLS success. You'll learn weight loss strategies, like mindful eating, that will help with any weight loss program. Finally, you'll explore what to expect from your presurgery medical evaluations as well as what to expect the first week or two after surgery.

Part 2

Preparing for Success by Taking Action

Preparation for WLS takes action. In this part of the book, you'll be asked to take a series of actions that move you toward WLS. It's imperative that you start an exercise program before surgery. The sooner you start exercising, the better your physical conditioning will be for surgery, so in the first chapter of part 2, you'll take action by developing an exercise program. Changing the way you eat is an important part of preparing for WLS. To change your eating habits, you first need to do a self-evaluation. In chapter 6 you'll evaluate your eating habits to identify problem eating behaviors. Problem eating behaviors include bad habits like making poor food choices as well as more serious problems like binge eating or emotional eating. Different types of problem eating behaviors require different actions. In chapter 7 you'll learn to substitute good eating habits for bad ones. *Cognitive restraint of eating* refers to how you use your thoughts to control eating. You'll take action in chapter 8 to improve your cognitive restraint of eating. Because it's not uncommon for people to use food to soothe difficult emotions, in chapter 9 you'll take action to control emotional eating. Social support from family and friends, as well as support from others who have had WLS, can help you make the transition from presurgery life to life after WLS. Taking action to mobilize your support team is the focus of chapter 10. Finally, in chapters 11 and 12 we'll look at what to expect from your presurgery appointments with the surgeon, psychologist, and registered dietitian, and what to expect the day of surgery and the first few weeks after surgery.

If you've decided the timing isn't right for surgery or decided against surgery, you'll find all but the last two chapters of this part helpful. Remember to look for this symbol ✻ at the start of each chapter section. If you see the symbol, it means the information in that section is as helpful for those like Rebecca, who are choosing conventional dieting, as it is for someone like Josie, who's preparing for surgery.

Chapter 5

Developing an Exercise Program

Good exercise habits will help you prepare for surgery, lose weight after surgery, and prevent weight regain. Many people find it difficult to exercise regularly, so a plan that takes into account your physical limitations and exercise history is important. Let's start our discussion with why exercise is important to metabolism.

WHY EXERCISE?

As we learned in chapter 1, exercise improves your basal metabolic rate (BMR), which increases your body's ability to burn calories. A recent study of weight-loss maintenance after WLS found that exercise was the most important factor in keeping weight off (Welch et al. 2010). Exercise isn't just helpful *after* WLS; many surgeons ask patients to lose weight *before* surgery. Being asked to lose about 10 percent of your total weight is a common requirement that exercise will help you meet. It's important to remember that exercise alone is usually not enough to produce weight loss. You'll also have to decrease the number of calories you take in. If you eat more calories, you'll counteract the advantage exercise gives you. Exercising before WLS improves your overall health. The healthier you are, the lower your risk for surgery complications and the faster you'll return to your normal activities after surgery.

While exercise is extremely beneficial, there's one thing exercise won't do for you: it won't prevent excess skin. If you lose a lot of weight and your skin has been overstretched, you'll have loose skin. Exercise will tone the muscles under the skin, but skin that has lost its elasticity won't bounce back, no matter how much toning you do before or after weight loss.

YOUR EXERCISE PLAN

There are four steps in developing an appropriate exercise plan, starting with consulting your doctor. Let's look at each step. Check each one as you complete it.

☐ Step 1: Consult Your Doctor

Because obesity causes serious health problems, the first step in developing an exercise plan is finding out what exercise is appropriate and safe for you. Mark's doctor told him to avoid stress on his knees, which could worsen his arthritis. Because Megan doesn't have any obesity-related health problems, her doctor told her she can choose any exercise she likes. Make an appointment with your doctor to talk about exercise. If you haven't already discussed WLS with your doctor, let her know your plans. It's always a good idea to take a list of questions with you anytime you go to the doctor. Important exercise questions to ask are:

- *How might my medical problems interfere with exercise?*

- *Are there any kinds of exercise that are not safe for me?*

- *What kind of exercise do you recommend?*

- *How long and how many times a week should I exercise in the beginning?*

Write your doctor's instructions in the following table:

My Doctor's Exercise Instructions

1. Suggested exercises:

2. Prohibited exercises and why:

3. Suggested duration of exercise:

4. How often per week:

☐ Step 2: Examine Your Past Exercise Experience

You can learn a lot about what kind of exercise program will work for you by examining what has and hasn't worked for you in the past. Answer the following questions about your past exercise experience.

My Past Exercise Experience

What Worked?

1. In the past what type of exercise did you enjoy?

2. Does it work best for you to exercise alone or with others?

3. If you exercise with others, which format works best?

   ☐ Class at the gym   ☐ An exercise buddy   ☐ Being part of a sports team

What Didn't Work?

1. What has stopped you in the past from starting an exercise program?

2. If you used to exercise but discontinued, why did you stop exercising?

3. Have you ever bought exercise equipment or joined a gym and never followed through? If you answered yes, why didn't you use your home equipment or gym membership?

What did you learn from looking at your past exercise experience? Mark realizes that the only time he was successful at exercising regularly was when he was part of a sports team. He stuck to his exercise plan when he played football and had a coach to motivate him, but he had little success on his own. Josie joined a gym several times and never made use of her membership. On the other hand, Josie did walk three times a week with a friend for more than a year. She realizes her lack of follow-through with her gym memberships stems from embarrassment. Josie believes that at the gym, she'd be judged by her weight, so the embarrassment stops her from exercising. In the next box, write what you learned from reviewing your exercise history.

My exercise history tells me:

☐ Step 3: Choose Appropriate Exercise

The good news about exercise is that exercise options abound, and it's rare that someone can't exercise at all. Along with your doctor's recommendations and what you learned from your exercise history, consider these exercise factors:

- *Calories:* How many calories does a particular exercise burn?

- *Frequency and exertion:* If you haven't been exercising regularly, start slowly. Starting with ten to fifteen minutes a day, five to six days a week, is better than going all out by spending ninety minutes at the gym from day one and rendering yourself unable to get out of bed the next morning. Slowly increase duration and difficulty of exercise over time.

- *Support:* If you have trouble getting motivated, an exercise buddy or class can help you get moving.

- *Professional help:* Physical therapists or personal trainers can tailor an exercise program for your physical limitations.

BURNING CALORIES

Different types of exercise expend different amounts of calories. Swimming, for example—which could be a good choice for someone with bad knees, like Mark—burns more calories per minute than walking. Look over the following chart to see how many calories some common types of exercise burn. You'll notice that the more you weigh, the more calories you burn, because in addition to benefiting from the exertion of the exercise itself, you are carrying extra weight, which requires additional exertion.

Activity (30 Minutes)	Weight of Person and Calories Burned			
	160 lb.	200 lb.	240 lb.	300 lb.
Jogging (5 mph)	326	361	434	542
Swimming (laps)	289	361	434	681
Aerobics (high impact)	254	318	381	477

Golfing (carrying clubs)	200	250	300	375
Aerobics (low impact)	180	227	272	338
Aerobics (water)	146	182	218	270
Bicycling (< 10 mph)	146	182	218	269
Yoga (gentle)	143	179	215	269
Walking (2 mph)	91	114	137	171
Walking (3 mph)	126	157	189	236
Weight lifting (free weight, Nautilus, or Universal type)	109	136	163	204

☐ Step 4: Develop Your Plan

Now it's time for you to commit to your own exercise plan. The best way to make a commitment is to develop a plan in writing. Considering your doctor's recommendations, fill out the exercise plan provided a little later. In addition to the standard types of exercise, like walking, using gym equipment, or taking an exercise class at the gym, lots of other options are available. For more ideas about types of exercise, check out this list:

- ◆ Walking in a pool
- ◆ Using exercise DVDs at home
- ◆ Doing yoga or tai chi
- ◆ Dancing
- ◆ Horseback riding
- ◆ Golfing
- ◆ Kickboxing
- ◆ Other: _____

Mark finds that exercising in a pool fits his doctor's recommendations. Because Mark knows he does best when he has someone to motivate him, he signs up for a water exercise class that meets three times a week and he meets with a personal trainer twice a week. Josie starts using an exercise bike four days weekly after work and signs up for a once-weekly yoga class for people with physical limitations. Megan, who has no real physical limitations, starts going to the gym with her mother three times a week to use the treadmill and lift weights. Many gyms give new customers a couple of free sessions with a personal trainer. Megan uses her sessions to learn how to use the equipment and develop a weight-lifting program she can follow. Now it's time for you to develop your plan. Remember, you'll have to make time to exercise, so be realistic. If you have a job that keeps you at the office late, don't plan on taking an exercise class at 5:00 p.m. Pick a schedule that works for your life. Try to plan to do some kind of exercise at least five days a week.

My Exercise Plan							
Day of Week	Sun	Mon	Tue	Wed	Thu	Fri	Sat
Type of Exercise							
Location							
Time of Day							
Duration							
Alone, or with a Buddy, Class, or Trainer							

✲ INCREASING YOUR DAILY ACTIVITY

Besides taking on a formal exercise program, increasing your physical activity during the day helps you burn calories and improve your health. The more active you are, the better condition you'll be in at the time of your surgery. While going up a few stairs can't replace your exercise plan, the more you move your body around, the better you'll feel, and it never hurts to burn a few extra calories. Next, check how you plan to increase your overall physical activity.

Ideas for Increasing Physical Activity Throughout the Day

☐ Take stairs instead of the elevator. If you have to go up more floors than you can handle, walk up one or two flights and then take the elevator.

☐ Park in distant parking spots.

☐ Use two-, five-, or ten-pound weights while watching TV to exercise your arms.

☐ Walk around the house during TV commercials.

☐ If you have a dog, take him for a daily walk. If you don't have one, offer to walk a neighbor's dog.

☐ Get a pedometer and challenge yourself to take an extra five hundred to one thousand steps per day each week.

☐ If you have a desk job, get up more often. Use the fax or copy machine that's farthest from your desk, or take the long way around when you head for lunch or the break room.

☐ Other ideas: _____

❊ SELF-MONITORING

Now that you have a plan, it's time to start self-monitoring. Self-monitoring, or keeping track of the exercise you do, has been shown to help with motivation (Carels et al. 2005). By keeping track of what exercise you do, you can see your progress. Slowly increasing the amount of exercise you do improves your body's conditioning.

Use the following exercise record to track your exercise. Write how much and what kind of exercise you did. In the last row, include any extra physical activities you did, like taking the stairs. If you don't like this log or prefer something more high tech, there are plenty of ways to keep exercise records online, plus there are applications for cell phones. You can even get fancy pedometers that produce an electronic record of when and how much you exercise. Pick the kind of record you think will work best for you. The important part is that you practice self-monitoring.

My Exercise Record

Day	Sun	Mon	Tue	Wed	Thu	Fri	Sat
Start time							
Type of exercise							
Time spent							
Extra activities							

*Include taking the stairs or other extra activities you engaged in.

STAYING MOTIVATED

Staying motivated can be difficult. Try these tips for keeping your exercise motivation high:

- Review your compelling goal frequently (at least twice a week).

- Make a commitment to exercise with a buddy. While you might not go to the gym on your own, you probably wouldn't stand up a friend who is counting on exercising with you.

- Reward yourself. Put money aside each week. If you stick to your exercise plan, use the money for something fun. On the other hand, if you don't follow your plan, donate the money to a charity, political party, or cause you dislike.

- Put your exercise plan someplace where you will see it regularly throughout the day. Post it on your bathroom door or refrigerator to remind you of the commitment you have made to your health and future.

WHAT'S NEXT?

Now that you've started to exercise, it's time to look at how and what you're eating. The action you'll take in the next three chapters will address problem eating, starting with evaluating the way you eat and what you need to change.

Chapter 6

Evaluating Problem Eating Behaviors

How you change your eating before WLS has a lot to do with how successful you'll be at changing your eating habits after your surgery. Problem eating is eating that interferes with success before and after surgery. It's rare for someone, obese or thin, to *never* engage in problem eating behaviors. Problem eating behaviors fall into two general categories:

- ◆ Bad eating habits
- ◆ Disordered eating

Bad eating habits include skipping breakfast or frequently eating fast food. More serious, *disordered eating* includes behaviors like binge eating. If disordered eating is severe enough, it can indicate an eating disorder. Even if disordered eating is something you only occasionally do and you don't have an eating disorder, all disordered eating must be resolved before surgery. The first step in resolving problem eating is identifying your bad eating habits. The second step is to determine whether you engage in disordered eating behaviors and could possibly have an eating disorder.

✻ BAD EATING HABITS

Abundant access to foods full of sugar, fat, and salt make bad eating habits easy to develop. In addition to which foods you eat, how you eat can lead to bad eating habits. A common example is eating too quickly. Look over this list of bad eating habits and check any you're aware of having:

- ☐ Skipping meals
- ☐ Eating while standing up in the kitchen rather than sitting at a table

☐ Snacking all day

☐ Eating out most of the time

☐ Eating in the car

☐ Eating junk food or fast food frequently (more than twice a week)

☐ Eating very quickly, for example, being the first one to finish a meal or eating so quickly you don't taste the food

☐ Drinking a lot of calories (having more than one drink a day that contains more than one hundred calories, such as soda, fruit juice, or energy drinks)

☐ Doing most of your eating in front of the TV or computer

☐ Always eating on the run

Sometimes bad eating habits are so ingrained in our lives that we aren't even aware of all the bad eating we engage in. A little later, you'll have the opportunity to do a baseline food log for one week. During that week, you may find additional bad habits you need to address. In the next chapter you'll learn to substitute good habits for the bad ones you discover now.

❊ DISORDERED EATING

Disordered eating is more than having bad eating habits. Sometimes, disordered eating is a symptom of an *eating disorder*, which is a psychological disorder involving abnormal eating behaviors that usually result from anxiety about weight and shape or an attempt to control unwanted emotions using food. Part of the definition of an eating disorder is that the disorder significantly interferes with your life. For example, bingeing every night in private rather than going out with friends, because you feel very guilty about how you eat and don't want anyone to see you eat, is disordered eating that's interfering with your life. On the other hand, bingeing occasionally—say, on Thanksgiving with the rest of the country—wouldn't be part of an eating disorder. This means it's possible to engage in some disordered eating without having an eating disorder. Disordered eating behaviors include:

♦ Binge eating

♦ Purging to get rid of food by vomiting or using a laxative

♦ Emotional eating

♦ Eating in your sleep

While only a mental health professional, like a psychologist who specializes in eating disorders, can tell for sure whether you have an eating disorder, if you engage in disordered eating regularly—say, once a week or more—you might have an eating disorder. Let's look at the kinds of eating disorders that are associated with obesity.

Eating Disorders

Eating disorders affect about one third of people who are obese. The most common type of eating disorder seen in people seeking WLS is *binge-eating disorder*. If your binge eating occurs several times a week or more, and it interferes with your life and causes you to feel guilty, disgusted, or depressed, you could have a binge-eating disorder (APA 2000). But remember, just because you binge sometimes doesn't necessarily mean you have an eating disorder. Some binges are triggered by bad habits, such as not eating all day and then being very hungry when you get home. That kind of binge is usually not part of an eating disorder.

What's a Binge?

The amount of food that constitutes a binge is somewhat subjective. In general, Americans tend to overeat. An example of overeating is eating a second helping of spaghetti or eating a large baked potato instead of a small one. A binge is more than overeating. A good rule of thumb for identifying a binge is to see if you follow one of these patterns:

- You eat twice as much or more than the average American would eat in a single two-hour period. An example might be eating two combination meals (burger, large fries, and large drink), when the average American would eat one combination meal.

- You eat so much you feel overfull to the point of discomfort.

While binge-eating disorder is the most common type of eating disorder seen in people seeking WLS, two other eating disorders, *bulimia nervosa* and *nighttime eating disorder*, are sometimes seen in people seeking WLS. Bulimia nervosa (often shortened to *bulimia*) is characterized by binge eating followed by *purging* behavior. Purging (usually by vomiting or using laxatives) is an attempt to compensate for the binge. Purging is unhealthy behavior before or after WLS. While the dangers of purging are less severe in people who are obese than in those who are underweight, it's possible to damage your throat by vomiting or to become dependent on laxatives.

Getting up in the middle of the night to eat, characteristic of nighttime eating disorder, can add calories to what you eat during the day. The three types of nighttime eating are:

- *Habit:* You're in the habit of eating in the middle of the night.

- *Insomnia:* You can't sleep, so you get up and have a snack.

- *Sleep disorder:* You're unaware that you're eating, and you have no memory of eating in the middle of the night.

The third type of nighttime eating is the most serious. Nighttime eating without awareness can be a symptom of a sleep disorder or a side effect of certain medications like Ambien (zolpidem) or Lunesta (eszopiclone) (Howell, Schenck, and Crow 2009).

While it's common to hear people talk about emotional eating, there's no eating disorder called "emotional eating disorder." Many people who have a binge-eating disorder or bulimia do binge and purge to get rid of unwanted emotions. Because emotional eating can cause problems before and after surgery, chapter 9 is devoted to resolving emotional eating. To determine your eating-disorder risk, answer the following eating-disorder screening questions:

Eating-Disorder Screening Questionnaire

Answer these questions based on your eating over the last six months.

Bingeing

1. Sometimes I eat a very large amount in a two-hour period.   ☐ Yes ☐ No

2. If others saw how much I ate, they would say it was a lot.   ☐ Yes ☐ No

3. I feel bad about myself after I eat large amounts of food.   ☐ Yes ☐ No

4. I eat large amounts of food more than once a week.   ☐ Yes ☐ No

Purging

5. I sometimes purge after I binge.   ☐ Yes ☐ No

6. I sometimes use a laxative to try to lose weight.   ☐ Yes ☐ No

Nighttime eating

7. I sometimes get up at night, eat, and return to bed.   ☐ Yes ☐ No

8. I sometimes find evidence that I've eaten in the middle of the night,
    such as wrappers or dirty plates, but have no memory of eating.   ☐ Yes ☐ No

Emotional eating

9. I often eat when I'm upset, anxious, angry, or sad.   ☐ Yes ☐ No

If you answered yes to one or more of the first four questions, you might meet the criteria for having binge-eating disorder. If you answered yes to question 5 or 6, you could have bulimia. Questions 7 and

8 are about nighttime eating. If you answered yes to question 8, you could have a sleep disorder that causes disordered eating. If you tend to eat when you feel strong unwanted emotions, you probably answered yes to question 9.

The good news is that eating disorders are very treatable. While sometimes self-help is enough to resolve an eating disorder, other times it's necessary to seek professional treatment from an *eating-disorder specialist*, often a psychologist who has specialized training in the evaluation and treatment of eating disorders. Binge-eating disorder, in particular, is responsive to self-help, but if you find that the suggestions in this part of the book or the self-help resources at the end of the book are not enough to resolve your binge eating, find an eating-disorder specialist to help you. If you think you have bulimia or a sleep disorder that involves eating while you're asleep, now is the time to seek a consultation with an eating-disorder specialist. If you do have an eating disorder and don't resolve it, the psychologist who evaluates you for WLS probably won't approve you for surgery.

SELF-EVALUATION

To change your behavior, you need to know exactly what you need to change, which requires collecting data. A *baseline food log* is a record of how you're eating now, before making changes. This log will give you the data you need to determine what eating behaviors need changing. Make copies of the following food log and keep a baseline food log for the next week.

Instructions for Keeping a Baseline Food Log:

Column 1: Record when and where you ate.

Column 2: Rate your hunger when you started to eat on a scale from 0 to 5, with 0 meaning no hunger and 5 meaning extremely hungry.

Columns 3 and 4: Record everything you eat or drink and approximate amounts.

Column 5: Note any purging, bingeing, overeating, or nighttime eating. If you think you ate too much but didn't binge, log your eating as overeating.

Column 6: Record your emotions before, during, and after you ate. For example, were you upset before you ate? Did you feel less anxious while you ate? Did you feel guilty after eating? Write in your own words how you felt.

Column 7: Note how you felt physically before and after you ate. For example, were you tired before you ate, or did you feel overly full after eating?

Column 8: For now, leave the trigger analysis section of the food log blank.

Baseline Food Log   Day: _____

Time and Location	Hunger Level 0–5	Food and Drink	Amount	Binged, Overate, Purged, or Ate at Nighttime	Emotions	Physical Feelings	Trigger Analysis
					Before: During: After:	Before: After:	
					Before: During: After:	Before: After:	
					Before: During: After:	Before: After:	
					Before: During: After:	Before: After:	
					Before: During: After:	Before: After:	
					Before: During: After:	Before: After:	

Analyzing Your Data

By now you probably have a week's worth of data from your log to analyze. Take these two steps:

1. Identify your problem eating behavior.

2. Determine what triggers your problem eating behavior.

Purging

If you're purging, share your food log with your eating-disorder specialist. It's important to determine what triggers your purging. The most common trigger for purging is overeating or bingeing, but there can be other triggers as well. Typically people feel anxious or upset after a binge and these emotions trigger purging, but this is not always the case. If your purging is in response to negative emotions about bingeing, the solution is to avoid the emotional trigger by eliminating binge eating. If, on the other hand, your purging is triggered by something else, you may need a different solution. Be sure to explore your purge triggers during your treatment with the eating-disorder specialist so you can eliminate these triggers.

Step 1: Identify your problem eating behavior. Look over your baseline food logs, check any of these problem eating behaviors you find, and note the frequency of each:

☐ Grazing or snacking all or most of the day; number of days: _____

☐ Grazing after dinner; number of days: _____

☐ Not eating early in the day, for example, skipping breakfast or skipping both breakfast and lunch; number of days: _____

☐ Standing in the kitchen while eating; number of times: _____

☐ Binge eating; number of binges: _____

☐ Overeating without bingeing; number of times: _____

☐ Eating out; number of times: _____

☐ Eating fast food; number of times: _____

☐ Eating in the car; number of times: _____

☐ Driving through the take-out lane so you can order your food and take it home without being seen by anyone; number of times: _____

☐ Eating in the middle of the night; number of times: _____

While the difference between overeating and bingeing is somewhat subjective, both are problem behaviors that need to be eliminated before surgery. How many times did you overeat or binge during the week? *Number of times I overate or binged in a week:* _____

Step 2: Determine your triggers. Many people engage in the problem eating behaviors just discussed, and most Americans, whether thin or obese, binge or overeat every once in a while. Review the following common reasons or triggers for problem eating behaviors. These are the triggers most often associated with bingeing, overeating, or eating high-calorie foods.

- *Physical:* Being overly hungry or tired

- *Emotional:* Trying to cope with anxiety, sadness, or other emotions using food

- *Sensory:* Seeing or smelling food

- *Opportunistic:* Being presented with a lot of food at a restaurant, potluck, or other setting where food is overly plentiful

- *Cognitive:* Thinking thoughts that lead to overeating—for example, thinking *I won't be able to eat this after WLS, so I should eat it now*

- *Habit:* Mindlessly eating out of habit while doing something else, like watching TV

You're almost ready to fill out the analysis section of your baseline food log, but before you do, let's look at a typical day on Josie's log to see her analysis.

Josie's Baseline Food Log   Day: Monday

Time and Location	Hunger Level 0–5	Food and Drink	Amount	Binged, Overate, Purged, or Ate at Nighttime	Emotions	Physical Feelings	Trigger Analysis
7:00 a.m. Kitchen	0	Coffee with sweetener	2 c.		Before: Just rushing to work During: Can't remember After: Can't remember	Before: Sleepy After: Awake	
10:00 a.m. My desk	0	Diet soda	1 can		Before: Felt good; hadn't eaten During: Too busy to remember After: Too busy	Before: Tired After: Better	
Noon My desk	2	Diet soda	1 can		Before: Felt good; hadn't eaten yet During: Too busy After: Anxious	Before: Tired After: Better	Started to feel hungry
1:00 p.m. My desk	3	100-cal. cookies Diet soda	2 pkgs. 1 can		Before: Felt good During: Distracted After: Felt okay after the first bag but then felt bad about eating more	Before: Need a nap After: Still tired	Was hungry and had the cookies in my desk; planned to eat one package but was still hungry

Time/Place	Hunger (0–5)	Food	Amount	Overate, binged?	Feelings (emotional)	Feelings (physical)	Situation/Thoughts
7:00 p.m. Steak house	5	Large Caesar salad Garlic bread Steak Potato with butter, sour cream, and bacon Ice cream sundae Iced tea	3 c. 2 pcs. 12 oz. Large 1/2 2 glasses	Overate, binged?	*Before:* Excited to see my friend *During:* Happy *After:* Good; had a good time	*Before:* A little tired *After:* Very full	Met a friend at my favorite restaurant and was very hungry; figured I saved my calories for dinner; shared ice cream with my friend; not sure if this was a binge or overeating
10:00 p.m. Home	0	Chips Cookies Diet soda	Large bag 6 1 can	Binged	*Before:* Felt a little bored *During:* Nothing *After:* Felt guilty after I realized how much I ate	*Before:* Didn't notice *After:* Kind of sick to my stomach	Home watching TV, planned to have a few chips; didn't realize I ate the whole bag until my favorite show was over; ate the cookies because I had already eaten the chips; seemed like TV habit eat while bored

Reviewing Josie's food log, here's what we learn about her eating habits that day:

- Didn't eat early in the day; drank caffeine instead.

- Used caffeine to fight fatigue. But she also gets anxious with excess caffeine.

- Felt good about not eating early in the day.

- Too busy and distracted at work to know how she felt.

- Binged after dinner, but unsure if dinner was a binge.

- Felt guilty after eating the chips and cookies.

- Felt overly full after dinner and sick after the TV binge.

- Typical of most people who are obese, Josie doesn't purge.

- Ate out. If we looked at her entire week, we'd see that Josie eats out often, about six times a week. About half the time, it's fast food.

- Has a habit of eating while watching TV.

- Was bored after she got home.

When Josie and I look at her log, we decide not eating early in the day is setting her up for being overly hungry. When Josie starts to eat breakfast and lunch, her hunger triggers disappear. As you'll learn in the next chapter, though common, hunger triggers are one of the easiest triggers to eliminate. Dinner started as overeating and ended in a binge in front of the TV. There's also a possibility that she overate out of boredom. Before she kept a baseline food log, Josie wasn't aware that she binged. In fact when we first met, she told me she didn't think she binged. Josie's experience is not unique. Without a baseline food log, many people are unaware of their exact eating habits. Josie thought of her evening eating in front of the TV as snacking, but when she analyzes her baseline food logs, she realizes that she binges at night if she's bored and watching TV. As we can see from her log, Josie doesn't do much emotional eating. Mark, on the other hand, does engage in emotional eating. When Mark and I look at his food log, the first thing we notice is that he eats when he's upset or angry, which usually means driving through the fast-food lane for fries and a burger or two. If you're eating in response to unwanted emotions, you'll have the opportunity to look at which emotions trigger eating and learn what to do about emotional triggers in chapter 9.

It's not uncommon to experience a combination of triggers. Let's look one more time at Josie's baseline food log to see how this works. There were two triggers at the restaurant: First, Josie experienced the *physical trigger* of hunger. Physical triggers are very powerful and hard to ignore. Josie's hunger trigger was paired with an *opportunity trigger*. Restaurants present us with a lot of food. In the presence of the strong physical trigger of hunger, it's the rare person who doesn't overeat when faced with an abundance of food. Josie's binge after dinner had different triggers. She discovered that she almost always snacked while watching TV, which means she started out with a *habit trigger*. She mindlessly got the chips out after turning on the TV. Her lack of attention to her behavior as she munched on the chips is typical of a habit binge. She was also bored, so that could also have triggered some of the eating. Once she realized she had eaten the entire bag of chips, Josie added a *cognitive trigger*, or thought trigger, thinking *I already blew it, so I may as well eat more.*

Look over your own food log. Choose a time when you overate or binged and answer these questions:

1. How did your hunger level affect your eating? _____

   _____

2. Did you feel very tired? Is it possible you were trying to feel more energetic by eating? _____

   _____

3. How did your emotional state affect your eating? _____

   _____

4. How did the smell or sight of food affect you? _____

   _____

5. How did your thinking affect your eating? _____

   _____

6. Did you eat out of habit, mindlessly? If so, when did you realize you were eating? _____

   _____

7. Did you experience more than one trigger at a time? If so, describe how one trigger led to another. _____

   _____

You have analyzed one problem eating episode. Now return to your log and fill out the analysis section for each day. Write what makes sense to you, what will help you understand your eating habits. If you ate three healthy meals and didn't overeat or binge one day, that's great! But take the opportunity to analyze that day, too. You can learn a lot from a good day.

Next, check the triggers you found on your baseline food log:

My Binge/Overeating Triggers

Physical:

☐ Hungry

☐ Tired

Emotional:

☐ Anxious or nervous

☐ Sad

☐ Angry

☐ Other emotions: _____

☐ *Sensory:* Seeing or smelling food

☐ *Opportunistic:* Being presented with a lot of food

☐ *Cognitive:* Thoughts that trigger my eating

_____

_____

_____

☐ *Habit:* Mindlessly eating out of habit

WHAT'S NEXT?

Now that you have identified what you need to change, the next three chapters will take you through resolving your problem eating behaviors. In the next chapter you'll have the opportunity to work on eliminating your bad habits by replacing the bad eating habits with good ones.

Chapter 7

Normalizing Your Eating Habits

In this chapter you'll take action to resolve problem eating due to bad habits by *normalizing*, which means forming good habits in place of the bad ones. Good eating habits can help you address some of your overeating and bingeing triggers, lose weight before WLS, and prepare you for eating after surgery. Normalizing is very effective for eliminating hunger, sensory, opportunistic, and habit triggers. While you work on developing good habits, it's helpful to have a tool that will provide you with nutritional information about the food you are eating. A nutritional tool will help you develop new eating habits that take into account nutritional value and portion sizes. And you'll find everything from nutritional applications for computer devices to low-tech pocket books that list calories and portion sizes to choose from. Pick a tool you're comfortable with and consult it each time you eat something new to make sure you're familiar with portion size, calories, and other nutritional information.

A Special Message If You're on a Medically Prescribed Diet

If you have a serious medical condition like kidney failure or another medical condition for which you have been prescribed a medical diet, it's important to follow the diet that was prescribed for you. You can probably follow most of the normalizing habits in this section, but some habits may not fit your medically prescribed diet. For example, some people on medically prescribed diets must limit protein. If this is the case for you, focusing on protein is a habit you do *not* want to develop. Check with your doctor if you have any questions about altering your medically prescribed diet.

DEVELOPING GOOD EATING HABITS

Each of the eight normalizing habits has a benefit. A good habit might resolve an overeating trigger, help you enjoy the food you eat, or help you prepare for surgery. Before we discuss each habit in detail, review the following chart to get an idea of the benefit of each habit. If you're dieting because your surgeon has told you to lose weight before surgery, or if you're like Rebecca and reading this chapter to help you lose weight with a conventional diet, these habits can also help you lose weight.

Eight Normalizing Habits	
Normalizing Habit	*Benefit*
Habit 1: Eat three meals a day on a schedule.	◆ Addresses hunger, sensory, and opportunistic triggers. ◆ Ensures that you get enough protein after surgery. ◆ Helpful for dieting. All healthy diets require three meals a day.
Habit 2: Eat only planned snacks.	◆ Addresses habit, sensory, and opportunistic triggers. ◆ If snacks are part of your weight loss program, planning snacks ensures that you don't eat too much or the wrong kind of food.
Habit 3: Eat small portions.	◆ Addresses habit and opportunistic triggers. ◆ Helpful for all diet plans.
Habit 4: Chew your food and avoid drinking calories.	◆ Ensures that food can fit through the small stomach opening after surgery. ◆ Helps maintain weight loss after surgery. ◆ Dieters who chew food feel more satisfied. ◆ Eliminates liquid calories, which are easily absorbed and can add hundreds of calories to your total calorie intake each day.
Habit 5: Give up caffeine, carbonation, and alcohol.	◆ Prepares you for post-WLS life.
Habit 6: Focus on protein.	◆ Addresses hunger trigger. ◆ Prepares for postsurgery protein focus.

Habit 7: Eat mindfully.	◆ Addresses all triggers.
	◆ Helps you enjoy food.
	◆ Especially helps dieters.
	◆ Helps you enjoy food after WLS.
Habit 8: Practice self-monitoring.	◆ Addresses all triggers.
	◆ Will help you adhere to the post-WLS food rules.
	◆ Dieters who self-monitor lose more weight and are more likely to keep the weight off.

Now let's look at each habit in detail to see how these habits can help you replace bad habits with good ones, address triggers, and prepare for surgery.

Habit 1: Eat Three Meals a Day on a Schedule

Before and after surgery, it's important to eat three meals a day. Before WLS, scheduling breakfast, lunch, and dinner prevents hunger triggers, which can set you up for sensory or opportunistic triggers. If you feel hungry, it's much harder to turn away when presented with the smell of home-baked cookies a coworker brings to work. Much of Josie's overeating results from skipping breakfast, and sometimes lunch, leaving her overly hungry at the end of the day. Eating three meals a day eliminates her hunger triggers. But it's not just eliminating the hunger trigger that makes eating three meals a day important. We learned in chapter 1 that eating sufficient protein after WLS is challenging. Skipping just one meal a day after surgery means losing one third of your protein for that day.

The best way to make sure you eat three healthy meals a day is to schedule your meals. Eating on the fly often means poor choices and hastily eaten food. It's also much harder to skip a meal if you adhere to a schedule.

Habit 2: Eat Only Planned Snacks

Post-WLS eating is usually limited to three meals a day to promote weight loss. But before surgery, in order to avoid hunger, planned snacks are a helpful tool. Planned snacks help reduce the size of meal portions and fend off hunger, sensory, and opportunistic triggers. Planning your snack ensures that the snack is healthy and doesn't become a binge. Before WLS, keeping snacks under 150 calories is a good rule. Because snacks are meant to get you to the next meal without getting too hungry, choose snacks that will satisfy you for at least two hours. Snacks that include protein and fiber will help with hunger between meals.

Satisfying Snack Ideas

Fruit and protein (examples):

◆ Small apple (77 calories) with a one-inch cube of cheddar cheese (69 calories)

◆ Small orange (45 calories) and 1/2 oz. (15 nuts) dry-roasted peanuts (83 calories)

◆ Your own example: (_____ calories)

High-protein snacks (examples):

◆ Almonds (20 nuts, 140 calories)

◆ Light string cheese (120 calories)

◆ One cup fat-free yogurt (100–137 calories)

◆ Your own example: (_____ calories)

Snacks to avoid:

◆ 100-calorie cookies or other "diet snacks" with little protein will probably leave you feeling hungry. These "diet snacks" are poor snack choices.

Habit 3: Eat Small Portions

Over time, Americans have increased servings to unhealthy sizes. We see this trend in restaurant food. Go to any restaurant and you'll likely get enough food for several people in one entrée. Familiarize yourself with how much food is in a healthy portion by checking out these examples:

◆ Pasta, rice, or potatoes: 1/2 cup

◆ Most meats: 4 ounces

◆ Cold cereal: 1 cup

◆ Fruits: small piece or 1/2 cup

◆ Most vegetables: 1 cup

Eating Out

Americans love to eat out. As long as you stay away from fast food, you can eat at most restaurants and still be true to your new eating plan. Try these ideas for healthy restaurant eating:

◆ Eat out twice a week or less.

◆ Use nutritional information to guide your order. Most restaurants will give you information on calories. Calorie comparisons provide good information for choosing your meal from a restaurant menu.

◆ Most restaurants serve portions that are too big. Get a take-home box *before* you eat, and put all but the portion of food you plan to eat in the box first.

◆ Split a meal with a friend.

◆ Go to restaurants that offer healthy menu choices or at least healthy substitutions. A restaurant that will give you veggies instead of fries is one to keep on your favorite restaurant list.

Habit 4: Chew Your Food and Avoid Drinking Calories

There are two reasons to focus on chewing. First, after surgery the opening to your stomach will be small. You must chew food very well so you can swallow without discomfort. Second, most of your calories should come from solid foods that require chewing. Mindlessly drinking hundreds of calories a day in sodas, energy drinks, juices, fancy coffee, or tea drinks loaded with cream and sugar is a common bad habit. Liquid calories are often empty calories that won't satisfy you. After WLS, drinking too many calories can lead to weight regain (the exception to this rule is the liquid protein drinks some doctors recommend after WLS to help boost your protein intake).

Drinking Calories

It's not hard to drink over 500 calories a day. Look at Megan's example, which follows, to see how she drinks 500 to 700 calories in one day.

Megan's typical day:

Time	Drink	Calories
9:00 a.m.	16-oz. sugared soda	230
11:00 a.m.	11 oz. of orange juice	150
1:00 p.m.	Frozen coffee drink	220
8:00 p.m.	16-oz. sugared soda	230
Total calories		830

Look over your baseline food log. Add up all the calories you drank each day. Next, write the number of calories you drank during the week. You can find calories for drinks in your nutritional tool (introduced at the beginning of this chapter) or at an online source (see the resources section in the back of this book).

Day	Mon	Tue	Wed	Thu	Fri	Sat	Sun
Calories							

How many calories did you drink in one week? _____

Habit 5: Give Up Caffeine, Carbonation, and Alcohol

Do not use caffeine; any kind of carbonated drink, including carbonated water; or alcohol after WLS. If you are accustomed to drinking carbonated, caffeinated, or alcoholic drinks, start changing these habits now.

- ◆ Carbonated bubbles can stretch a small stomach, make you feel sick, and cause gas.

- ◆ Caffeine is irritating to a surgically altered stomach. If you currently drink more than one caffeinated drink a day, it's best to slowly switch to decaffeinated drinks so you don't get a caffeine withdrawal headache. Cut your caffeine by a little each week until you've eliminated it from your diet. If you drink decaf coffee or tea with sugar, now is the time to switch to a sugar substitute. It's okay to drink decaffeinated coffee or tea after surgery, so slowly switching over beforehand will allow you to enjoy decaffeinated, noncarbonated drinks without sugar after surgery.

- Alcohol contains empty calories, and if you have a type of WLS that causes malabsorption of nutrients, like RNYGB, alcohol can be dangerous after surgery. Your body's ability to metabolize alcohol changes after WLS, and it's possible for you to become drunk on a small amount. Before you think this is a good party strategy, understand that this means you can experience alcohol toxicity or become alcohol dependent more easily. So it's best to get into the habit now of having dinner without that glass of wine. If you find you can't stay away from alcohol, before surgery seek professional help from a mental health professional who has experience in alcohol dependency or abuse.

Habit 6: Focus on Protein

After WLS, most of the calories you consume should come from lean protein sources like meat, eggs, or low-fat yogurt. Depending on your type of surgery, you'll have to eat at least 70 grams of protein while losing weight and then 60 to 90 grams a day after that for the rest of your life (Aills et al. 2008). Eating this much protein is difficult when you have a small stomach that holds only a few ounces, so filling up on food that doesn't contain protein means you won't get enough protein. By focusing on protein, you'll develop a good postsurgery habit and, because protein takes longer to digest, probably feel more satisfied after you eat. But focusing on protein doesn't mean eating only protein and not eating vegetables, fruits, or grain-based foods like pasta. Before surgery you can probably eat a small serving of fruits or vegetables at each meal in addition to protein, while limiting food like bread, pasta, rice, or potatoes to a small amount once or twice a day. If you eat a variety of healthy foods while making sure to eat protein at each meal, you will probably get the nutrients you need before surgery. Follow these tips for making healthy food choices:

- Eat lean protein, like skinless chicken breast, tofu, eggs, or beans, at every meal.

- Eat low-fat foods.

- Limit carbohydrates like rice or bread to one or two small servings a day.

- When you eat carbohydrates, make sure they're complex carbohydrates. For example, eat whole grains instead of foods made with white flour.

- Eat less processed food, which means eating food that's closer to the way it developed in nature.

- As much as possible, limit foods that combine fat and sugar.

- Eat whole fruit, which has natural fiber, but avoid fruit juice.

- Choose fruits that are lower in sugar. Use your nutritional guide to learn which fruits are best.

- Eat vegetables without the addition of butter or sauces.

- Eat healthy food you like.

- Read food labels.

Reading Food Labels

Getting in the habit of reading food labels can help you determine how much protein is in food. Look at the following sample food label. Not only can we see that there are more than 10 grams of protein, but we can also see how much sugar, sodium (salt), fat, and calories are in this yogurt (this is just a sample; don't assume that all yogurt has the same nutrition facts).

Nutrition Facts: Sample Yogurt

Calories 250		(1045 kJ)
		% Daily Value
Total Fat	2.7 g	4%
Sat. Fat	1.7 g	9%
Cholesterol	10 mg	3%
Sodium	142 mg	6%
Total Carbohydrates	46.8 g	16%
Dietary Fiber	0 g	0%
Sugars	46.7 g	
Protein	10.7 g	
Calcium	372.4 mg	
Potassium	477.8 mg	

Daily requirements for protein, calcium, and potassium are not always reported on food labels, as these requirements can differ depending on age and health status. Consult with your doctor to find out how much calcium and potassium you need. After surgery, you will need more protein than a person with a normal digestive system.

Habit 7: Eat Mindfully

Mindfulness is about observing and focusing on one thing at a time. Mindful eating means paying attention, slowing down, and really enjoying what you eat. Eating quickly or multitasking while eating leads to overeating and interferes with enjoyment. Eating mindfully will help you with all of your overeating or bingeing triggers.

Eating Mindfully

Try these mindful eating behaviors (check those you plan to try):

- ☐ Slow down.
- ☐ Notice the taste and texture of food.
- ☐ Eat while sitting down at a table.
- ☐ Enjoy the smell and appearance of the food before you eat it.
- ☐ Put your fork or spoon down in between each bite.
- ☐ Chew your food at least twenty times before swallowing.
- ☐ Use nice tableware and cloth napkins.
- ☐ Make mealtime a time to bond with family or friends. Stop eating once in a while and really listen to the other person; use the meal as an opportunity to connect.

Habit 8: Practice Self-Monitoring

By using your baseline food log, you already have experience with self-monitoring. Monitoring what you eat using a food log is the best way to change your eating habits and stay on track. People who make self-monitoring part of their daily routine tend to lose more weight and keep the weight off. This is true for people who lose weight with both conventional dieting and WLS. Before surgery, self-monitoring can help you eliminate bad eating habits or disordered eating. After WLS self-monitoring will help you keep track of protein and troubleshoot any problem eating you might experience.

SELF-MONITORING LOG

Now that you know about the eight normalizing habits, it's time to make the habits part of your daily routine. The best way to do that is with the self-monitoring food log. Make copies of the log at the end of this chapter, or if you prefer, you can use one of the many electronic self-monitoring logs now available (see below, "Picking an Electronic Self-Monitoring Log"). Plan to self-monitor from now until at least one year after surgery. While this might seem like a long time, remember that research has shown that people who practice self-monitoring are more likely to lose weight and keep it off (Carels et al. 2005). And as we will learn in part 3 of this book, any time you run into problems after surgery, like weight regain or protein deficiency, the first thing to do is start self-monitoring again.

Picking an Electronic Self-Monitoring Food Log

Many electronic self-monitoring logs are available that produce weekly charts for adherence to an eating plan, plus there are easy-to-use self-monitoring log applications for cell phones. It's a good idea to use the self-monitoring log in this book for at least a week or two first, so you know what to look for. If you choose to go electronic, make sure your log allows you to:

- Record what you ate and when you ate it.

- Record problem eating behaviors like overeating or skipping meals.

- Troubleshoot solutions to problem eating behaviors.

- Pick a log that includes a place to record exercise, if you don't want to keep a separate exercise log.

Take the following steps in using a self-monitoring log.

Self-Monitoring Step 1

The first step is to create your eating schedule by writing when you plan to eat each meal or snack in column 1 of the self-monitoring food log at the end of this chapter. A good rule of thumb is to space your meals and snacks about three to four hours apart. If you're not eating snacks, space your meals about five hours apart. Some surgeons prefer that patients stop eating snacks before surgery, so if you've seen a surgeon and been given this advice, drop down to three meals a day.

Self-Monitoring Step 2

Now it's time to start using your self-monitoring food log.

Instructions for Using the Self-Monitoring Food Log:

Column 1: Indicate whether you ate a meal or a snack. If your eating was unplanned, note what time you ate.

Column 2: Record what you ate and drank, and the amount.

Column 3: Record whether you ate mindfully. This means you paid attention to eating and really tasted your food. This also means not watching TV, working at your computer, or doing other tasks while you eat.

Column 4: Record problem-eating behaviors like purging, bingeing, or overeating. Some people can stop bingeing or purging by practicing the eight normalizing habits. After four weeks of following the normalizing habits, if you find you're still bingeing once a week or more, or purging, seek professional help.

Column 5: Track how you felt emotionally before, during, and after your meal or snack. This information is very important for determining if you do any emotional eating. We'll look at eliminating emotional eating in chapter 9.

Column 6: See "Self-Monitoring Step 3," which follows.

Finally, at the bottom of the log, write how much and what type of exercise you did. If you prefer to keep two logs, you can continue your exercise record from chapter 5.

Self-Monitoring Step 3

Once you have logged your food, eating problems, and other information, you can fill out the last column. First check whether you adhered to your plan. In other words, did you practice the eight normalizing habits, or avoid emotional eating or other problem eating behavior? If you missed your scheduled meal or snack by more than thirty minutes, you didn't adhere to your eating schedule. If you didn't adhere to your plan, it's time to determine what happened and find a solution. For example, maybe you didn't eat within thirty minutes of your scheduled time and got overly hungry, or maybe you overate at a barbecue because the food looked so good. For each problem, write what happened. If you skipped a meal, why did you skip? Did you get up too late to have breakfast or get so busy at work you lost track of time? Below your description of what happened, write your solution for avoiding the problem next time. Maybe you need to set your alarm for an earlier time so you'll have time for breakfast, or set an alarm to remind you when to eat lunch. As you go through the next three chapters, you'll learn additional solutions for eating problems. Continue to self-monitor as you add these solutions to your skill set.

Self-Monitoring Food Log   Day: _____

Schedule	Food/Amount	Ate Mindfully	Problem Eating	Emotions	Adhered to Plan/Solutions
☐ Meal ☐ Snack ☐ Unplanned eating Time: _____		☐ Yes ☐ No		Before: During: After:	☐ Yes ☐ No If no, what happened? _____ Solution: _____
☐ Meal ☐ Snack ☐ Unplanned eating Time: _____		☐ Yes ☐ No		Before: During: After:	☐ Yes ☐ No If no, what happened? _____ Solution: _____
☐ Meal ☐ Snack ☐ Unplanned eating Time: _____		☐ Yes ☐ No		Before: During: After:	☐ Yes ☐ No If no, what happened? _____ Solution: _____

☐ Meal
☐ Snack
☐ Unplanned eating

Time: _____

☐ Yes
☐ No

Before:
During:
After:

☐ Yes ☐ No
If no, what happened? _____
_____

Solution: _____
_____

☐ Meal
☐ Snack
☐ Unplanned eating

Time: _____

☐ Yes
☐ No

Before:
During:
After:

☐ Yes ☐ No
If no, what happened? _____
_____

Solution: _____
_____

Time spent exercising: _____   Type of exercise: _____

WHAT'S NEXT?

The way we think has a lot to do with how we eat. Thoughts like *I already ate too much, so I may as well eat more* or *Drinking one soda won't hurt me* cause problems before and after surgery. In the next chapter we'll address eating problems by developing cognitive restraint of eating.

Chapter 8

Developing Cognitive Restraint of Eating

Cognitive refers to thoughts, and cognitive restraint of eating (CRE) is how much your thoughts help you control how and what you eat. People with high CRE tend to lose more weight and experience less weight regain after WLS than people with low CRE (Welch et al. 2010). In this chapter you'll learn to change cognitive triggers into thoughts that build high CRE.

 ## COGNITIVE TRIGGERS VS. COGNITIVE RESTRAINT

Even if you aren't always aware of the exact thought, a thought always precedes eating (Beck 2007). A cognitive trigger is a thought that leads to eating too much food or the wrong kind of food. An example of a cognitive trigger is *I skipped breakfast, so I can have a candy bar*. CRE thoughts help you control your eating by triggering restraint. And this is true for conventional dieting or WLS. Thoughts that build CRE eliminate cognitive triggers by:

- Supporting your goals for better health and appearance

- Reminding you of the consequences of eating that sabotage your goals

Consider the CRE thought *My health is more important than the temporary pleasure of chocolate. If I eat the chocolate, it'll interfere with my weight loss and I'll feel bad about myself later.* This thought reinforces your goal to improve your health and reminds you of the consequences of ignoring that goal. CRE can help you with many kinds of eating problems. Look over the following list, and check the behaviors and beliefs you need help with:

- ☐ Eating three meals

- ☐ Staying away from sweets and treats

- ☐ Controlling portion sizes

- ☐ Staying away from fast food or eating out too often

- ☐ Eliminating soda, caffeine, or alcohol

- ☐ Keeping the self-monitoring food log

- ☐ Believing you can successfully lose weight

- ☐ Believing your health is worth changing the way you eat

- ☐ Other: _____

You've probably practiced your cognitive triggers over the years. Building CRE is about practice too. It takes practice and commitment to change your thinking, but it's possible. Here are the three steps to building a high CRE:

1. Understand the eleven common cognitive triggers.

2. Identify your cognitive triggers.

3. Change your cognitive triggers into thoughts that build CRE.

Understand Common Cognitive Triggers

Cognitive triggers are thoughts that lead to sabotaging behaviors like eating too much or believing you'll never be successful at losing weight. Examine the following eleven common obesity-related cognitive triggers and place a check mark in the box next to those you think you use.

Eleven Common Cognitive Triggers	
Type	*Example*
☐ Reward/celebration trigger	*I work hard and deserve a treat.* *It's my birthday (or Thanksgiving, Christmas, or Hanukkah), I can eat whatever I want.*
☐ Bad-day trigger	*This was the day from hell! I deserve to eat _____!* *I'll feel better if I eat _____.*
☐ "This is the last time" trigger	*I won't be able to eat this after my surgery, so I should eat it now.* *After today, I won't eat _____.*
☐ "I already blew it" trigger	*I ate the chips, so I may as well eat _____.* *I blew it and overate at lunch, so it doesn't matter if I overeat at dinner.*
☐ "I'll make up for it later" trigger	*I can eat this now and skip dinner.* *I'll eat what I want now and start eating healthy tomorrow.*
☐ "I saved the calories" trigger	*I haven't eaten all day, so I can eat.* *I didn't eat breakfast, so I can eat more at dinner.*
☐ Self-blame trigger	*If I were a stronger person, I would be able to lose weight.* *It's my fault I'm fat.*
☐ "It's not fair, other people do it" trigger	*It's not right that other people can eat what they want.* *Other people don't keep food logs; why should I?*
☐ "Life got in the way" trigger	*I don't have time to eat breakfast.* *Eating healthy is expensive.*
☐ Should/shouldn't trigger	*I should only eat healthy foods.* *I shouldn't eat dessert.*
☐ "I'm already defeated" trigger	*I've never been able to lose weight, so what does it matter what I eat?* *I'll never keep the weight off, so I may as well enjoy myself.*

Let's look at each of these triggers in detail to learn more about them, starting with the reward/celebration trigger.

REWARD/CELEBRATION TRIGGER

Let's face it: food is rewarding. You may have grown up in a family that used food as a reward; lots of us did. If you did, reward and food may be linked in your mind. You think *reward* and food comes to mind, so you may find that you frequently reward yourself with food. Mark puts it this way: "One of my earliest memories is of my grandmother baking my favorite cookies when I did well in school, and my mom continued that tradition by baking whenever anything good happened in the family. When I consider rewarding myself, a trip to the bakery comes to mind!"

Alternative Ways to Reward Yourself

There are lots of ways to reward yourself without food. From this list, check alternative rewards you plan to try (add at least two rewards you like that aren't listed):

☐ Getting time by yourself

☐ Reading a chapter in a favorite book

☐ Calling a loved one

☐ Having a cup of decaffeinated tea and listening to your favorite music

☐ Having a pedicure or manicure

☐ Buying or picking flowers

☐ Other reward:

☐ Other reward:

Like rewards and food, celebrations and food go together. This wasn't a big problem when food was scarce. In those days people saved "special food" for a few occasions a year. Now, instead of getting a small piece of cake once or twice a year, you can celebrate with cake every day. Some employers even have monthly birthday celebrations with cake for everyone. While this might not seem like a big deal, if you add this to all the other celebrations people observe, there's probably something to celebrate with cake or other special foods once a week or more. Next, describe the last time you used food as a reward or to celebrate something.

I used food to reward myself or celebrate:

BAD-DAY TRIGGER

As we'll discuss more thoroughly in chapter 9, many people use food to soothe difficult emotions. It's not uncommon to feel better as you eat. Unfortunately food is a poor way to soothe emotions, because on top of hurting your health, you'll probably feel worse after eating (which can lead to more eating). For this reason, one of the strongest alternative thoughts to a bad-day trigger is *I might feel better while I'm eating, but I'll feel worse afterward*. In chapter 9 we'll explore feeling better without food, but for now, start noticing whether you reach for food when you feel bad. Have you ever used food when you were having a bad day? Next, describe when you last used food in response to a bad day.

I used food to cope with a bad day:

"THIS IS THE LAST TIME" TRIGGER

This powerful trigger is often prompted by the decision to have WLS. When Mark first brings me his food log, he hands it to me and says, "I know I won't be able to eat ice cream after surgery, so I figure this is my last opportunity to enjoy my favorite flavors." Mark's thoughts interfere with his preparation for WLS, and he is actually eating ice cream more often than before he decided to have WLS. Let's look at the consequences of the "this is the last time" trigger:

- ◆ Interferes with WLS preparation and will sabotage you if your surgeon requires you to diet and lose weight before WLS.

- ◆ Makes food very important. If you think *This is the last time I can ever have ice cream*, it means ice cream is something very important. No one wants to be deprived of something important.

- ◆ Leads to the post-WLS thought *I'll have this just one more time*.

Since starting to prepare for WLS, have you used the "this is the last time" trigger? If you have had this thought, describe next how the thought affected your eating.

The "this is the last time" trigger affected me by:

"I ALREADY BLEW IT" TRIGGER

You have probably experienced this common diet-sabotaging thought, guaranteed to stop any diet in its tracks. What was the consequence of this thought for you in the past? For Mark, this trigger always means an end to his dieting. For Megan this thought results in the end of her diet, coupled with poor self-esteem, because she combines this thought with a self-blame thought: I blew it, and I'm a failure. Next, describe how this common thought trigger has affected you.

In the past, the "I already blew it" trigger led to:

"I'LL MAKE UP FOR IT LATER" TRIGGER

Related to the "I already blew it" trigger, this cognitive trigger usually goes something like this:

◆ Making up for the extra calories means not eating or not eating enough, which leads to hunger.

◆ Hunger leads to overeating and the "I already blew it" trigger, and the cycle repeats until you give up.

"I SAVED THE CALORIES" TRIGGER

This is a sneaky thought that can make you think you're doing well. *I saved calories, so I can eat _____* might seem logical, but it usually ends in overeating or eating the wrong food, and it often triggers the "I already blew it" cycle mentioned previously.

SELF-BLAME TRIGGER

Sometimes people think self-blame will lead to weight loss, but it never does. Self-blame is a put-down that doesn't lead to behavior change, but often leads to poor self-esteem and self-loathing, which can trigger emotional eating. Self-blame is different from taking responsibility. A thought that promotes responsibility is not a personal put-down, but rather a review of facts and remedy. Consider the following two thoughts:

◆ *I stopped logging what I ate, which resulted in my eating unhealthy food and gaining two pounds. Now it's time to take responsibility by restarting my food log and getting back on track.*

◆ *I'm a loser who will never lose weight.*

Which thought do you think would lead to a positive behavior change? Which thought leads to feeling bad but not changing your behavior? The first thought is a CRE thought that emphasizes taking responsibility by outlining what happens and what action to take. The second thought can lead to emotional eating.

"IT'S NOT FAIR, OTHER PEOPLE DO IT" TRIGGER

Thinking *It's not fair* or *Other people do it* rarely leads to positive changes. It's true that some people can eat more than others without gaining weight. While this is just a fact of biology (not fairness), if you think it's unfair, you may eat out of rebellion. The "other people do it" part of this trigger can be particularly problematic after WLS. Almost every week, as I teach my WLS class, I hear, "I have a friend who lost 120 pounds with WLS, and she eats _____, so why do I have to give up _____?" It's true; plenty of people who've had WLS don't follow the postsurgery food rules. And while it's also true that a few people can "get away with" eating outside of rules, most will regain weight over time.

"LIFE GOT IN THE WAY" TRIGGER

In the busy lives most of us lead, this trigger is often about time: I didn't have time to cook, I was too busy to stop for lunch, and so on. Also in this category is a thought I often hear: It's too expensive to eat healthy. This thought, which discounts the cost of obesity, leads Mark to eat a lot of cheap, unhealthy fast food.

Is It Really More Expensive to Eat Healthy Food?

While it can be expensive to eat healthy, it doesn't have to be. In general, fast food and junk food are less expensive per calorie, but a lot of cheap food is high in calories, fat, and sugar. Try buying nutrient-rich, in-season foods (and local, when possible) and decreasing portion size. In doing so, you can stretch your grocery dollars. Add up what you spend in prescription costs for obesity-related conditions like diabetes, plus the deductible or co-pay for doctor visits to monitor your health problems, and you may find that you come out ahead.

SHOULD/SHOULDN'T TRIGGER

This trigger is a little tricky, because on the surface, should/shouldn't thoughts seem helpful. But just telling yourself you should or shouldn't do something usually backfires. How many times have you thought, *I shouldn't eat* _____, as you put the food in your month, or *I should start my diet* as you reach for seconds? What happens when you think, *I shouldn't eat chocolate?* Does it make you want to eat more chocolate? Megan puts it this way: "As soon as I think I shouldn't eat a candy bar, all I want to do is eat the candy bar." So despite the veneer of logic this trigger has, it's much better to think, *If I eat breakfast, I won't overeat at lunch* rather than *I should eat breakfast.* The good thing about should/shouldn't triggers is that they're easy to recognize. Anytime the words "should," "shouldn't," or "have to" are in a thought, it's a should/shouldn't trigger.

"I'M ALREADY DEFEATED" TRIGGER

This might also be called the "I give up" trigger. If you think you can't be successful with your weight loss plan, you'll never follow it. Thinking you're already defeated easily leads to *I may as well eat what I want.* This trigger is often paired with self-blame, as in *I'm a weak person; I'll never be able to lose weight.*

COMBINING COGNITIVE TRIGGERS

Cognitive triggers often trigger each other, resulting in a cascade of triggers that can overtake our thinking. Let's look at Megan's example, which follows, to see how this works:

Megan thinks, *I'm such a fat slob* → feels bad about herself → eats a candy bar to feel better → thinks, *I blew it; I shouldn't have eaten the candy bar* → thinks, *I'll eat what I want today and make up for it tomorrow* → next day skips breakfast and lunch → is very hungry after school → overeats → *I'm such a loser; I blew it again.*

How many cognitive triggers do you see in Megan's example? Hint: there are at least four.

❈ Identify Your Cognitive Triggers

You probably now have a good understanding of each common cognitive trigger and are starting to get a good idea of what cognitive triggers you use. Now it's time to use the information you've been compiling in your self-monitoring logs to learn more about your cognitive triggers using the following cognitive trigger log. But before you fill out the log, let's look at part of Josie's cognitive trigger log. Josie reviews her self-monitoring logs, and each time she finds a record of deviating from her plan or engaging in problem eating behaviors, she tries to recall what she was thinking before she ate. Josie comes up with the following thoughts, which she writes in her log. Review Josie's thoughts and write in the "Cognitive Trigger" column which of the eleven cognitive triggers you think Josie was using.

Josie's Cognitive Trigger Log		
Day/Time	My Thoughts	Cognitive Trigger
Mon./7:00 a.m.	I don't have time for breakfast.	
Mon./Dinner	I didn't eat all day; I can eat what I want tonight.	
Mon./After Dinner	I ate the chips, so screw it.	

Which triggers did you come up with? When Josie and I looked over the thoughts in her log, we came up with the "life got in the way," "I saved the calories," and "I already blew it" triggers. It's common to have favorite cognitive triggers. Josie finds that she is fond of the first two triggers. Mark tends to use the "this is the last time," bad-day, and "it's not fair, other people do it" triggers more than the others. Megan often uses the self-blame trigger, which starts a chain of other triggers.

Now it's time to review your self-monitoring food logs. Look at the days you deviated from your plan or engaged in problem eating behaviors, and think back to right before you ate. What were you thinking? That's the thought to use in your cognitive trigger log, which follows. For each thought, write the cognitive trigger you were using (for now, leave the CRE column blank; we'll come back to it).

My Cognitive Trigger Log			
Day/Time	My Thoughts	Cognitive Trigger	Alternative CRE Thought

✳ CHANGE YOUR COGNITIVE TRIGGERS INTO THOUGHTS THAT BUILD CRE

Once you have identified your cognitive triggers, it's time to change your trigger thoughts to CRE thoughts. Let's look at the should/shouldn't trigger to see how to change a trigger into a thought that builds CRE. Should/shouldn't triggers are very common, so they are good practice thoughts. You probably found at least one should trigger when you looked at your cognitive triggers. Changing the "should" or "shouldn't" to thoughts that reinforce your goals and remind you of the consequences of your eating builds your CRE. Practice changing each should thought to a CRE thought:

Example: *I should eat breakfast.* →

Eating breakfast will help me stay on track with my plan to lose weight before WLS by keeping hunger at bay so that I don't overeat at lunch.

I shouldn't eat sweets. →

_____

_____

I should start my self-monitoring food log. →

_____

_____

I should eat more vegetables. →

_____

_____

How did you do? Were you able to change the should/shouldn't triggers into thoughts that reinforced your weight-loss goals or changed your beliefs about losing weight? Don't worry if you found it difficult to change the thoughts. Most of us have spent years practicing cognitive triggers, so it takes time and lots of practice to change these thoughts. Let's practice some more by changing the eleven common cognitive trigger examples we reviewed at the beginning of the chapter. To get you started, the first thought under each cognitive trigger has been changed into a CRE thought. These are examples only; you might come up with even better CRE thoughts. Practice on the second example by rewriting each cognitive trigger into a CRE thought.

Eleven Common Cognitive Triggers

Type	Example Trigger Thoughts	New CRE Thoughts
Reward/ celebration trigger	1. I work hard and deserve a treat. 2. It's my birthday (or Thanksgiving, Christmas, or Hanukkah); I can eat whatever I want.	1. I work hard and deserve to be healthy, and the treat won't help me be healthy. I can treat myself with something else. 2. CRE thought: _____ _____
Bad-day trigger	1. This was the day from hell! I deserve to eat _____! 2. I'll feel better if I eat _____.	1. This was a difficult day, but eating food that's bad for me will just make the day worse and sabotage my weight loss. 2. CRE thought: _____ _____
"This is the last time" trigger	1. I won't be able to eat this after my surgery, so I should eat it now. 2. After today I won't eat _____.	1. Giving up sweets is worth extending my life by getting my diabetes under control. It'll get easier the longer I keep from eating sweets. 2. CRE thought: _____ _____
"I already blew it" trigger	1. I ate the chips, so I may as well eat _____. 2. I blew it and overate at lunch. It doesn't matter if I overeat at dinner.	1. I ate the chips, but I can get back on track right now. 2. CRE thought: _____ _____

Type	Example Trigger Thoughts	New CRE Thoughts
"I'll make up for it later" trigger	1. I can eat this now and skip dinner. 2. I'll eat what I want now and start eating healthy tomorrow.	1. I want to eat this, but if I wait and distract myself, probably the urge to eat it will go down and I'll stay on my plan. 2. CRE thought: _____ _____
"I saved the calories" trigger	1. I haven't eaten all day, so I can eat _____. 2. I didn't eat breakfast, so I can eat more at dinner.	1. Not eating all day is unhealthy. I'll feel better about myself if I eat a healthy dinner without. 2. CRE thought: _____ _____
Self-blame trigger	1. If I were a stronger person, I would be able to lose weight. 2. It's my fault I'm fat.	1. It's about practice, not strength. I can learn to lose weight. 2. CRE thought: _____ _____
"It's not fair, other people do it" trigger	1. It's not right that other people just eat what they want to eat. 2. I know people having the lap band who say it's okay to drink soda.	1. People differ in how much they can eat. I will eat the right amount of food for my body to be healthy. 2. CRE thought: _____ _____
"Life gets in the way" trigger	1. I don't have time to eat breakfast. 2. Eating healthy is expensive.	1. Being unhealthy takes up a lot of time in doctor's appointments and trips to the pharmacy. It makes more sense to make time to improve my health by making breakfast the night before or getting up a little earlier. 2. CRE thought: _____ _____

Should/shouldn't trigger	1. *I should only eat healthy foods.* 2. *I shouldn't eat dessert.*	1. *It's not about "should" or "shouldn't"; it's about what's healthy for my body and reaching my goals.* 2. CRE thought: _____ _____
"I'm already defeated" trigger	1. *I've never been able to lose weight, so what does it matter what I eat?* 2. *I'll never keep the weight off, so I may as well enjoy myself.*	1. *Losing weight is difficult, but I'm working on the skills I need to successfully lose weight with WLS.* 2. CRE thought: _____ _____

Now it's time to rewrite your own trigger thoughts. Return to your cognitive trigger log and fill in the "Alternative CRE Thought" column. For the next week, review your self-monitoring food log, and fill out a cognitive trigger log each time you deviate from your plan or engage in a problem eating behavior. It's not necessary to continue using the cognitive trigger log unless you want to. After the first week, you can put your CRE thought right in your self-monitoring food log in the "Adhered to Plan/Solutions" column if your eating problem was due to a cognitive trigger. Over time you'll find that analyzing and rewriting cognitive triggers will lead to improved CRE. As your CRE thinking replaces cognitive triggers, you'll find it easier to follow your plan and avoid problem eating behaviors.

WHAT'S NEXT?

There are probably few people, thin or obese, who haven't eaten in response to emotion at some time. While not every obese person engages in frequent emotional eating, emotional eating is a common problem. Regularly eating in response to emotions can lead to problems like binge eating. Even if you think you don't engage in frequent emotional eating, complete the activities in the next chapter. You may be surprised to find that you're an emotional eater.

Chapter 9

Controlling Emotional Eating

Eating can be soothing, so it's not surprising that some people eat when experiencing sadness, anxiety, or other unwanted emotions. But eating can also be a response to happiness. In this chapter we'll look at the emotional eating cycle and how to deal with emotions without food. While emotional eating is not usually associated with a psychological disorder, sometimes this behavior is tied to a disorder like major depressive disorder, generalized anxiety disorder, or an eating disorder. We'll start our discussion with the emotional eating cycle.

❖ THE EMOTIONAL EATING CYCLE

It's normal to take action to decrease unwanted emotions. If a particular action works, like eating, we'll probably try that action again. And the truth is many people find that eating decreases unwanted emotions temporarily. Common unwanted emotions that can trigger eating include:

- ◆ Sadness
- ◆ Hopelessness
- ◆ Anxiety or nervousness
- ◆ Anger or frustration
- ◆ Guilt or shame
- ◆ Loneliness
- ◆ Boredom

Happy Eating

Happiness can trigger emotional eating. If you find yourself eating when you're happy, it's probably related to the reward/celebration cognitive trigger we discussed in chapter 8. Work on changing your thinking about happiness. There are lots of ways to respond to happiness. Make a list of happy responses that don't involve food, and remind yourself that eating in response to happiness leads to unwanted emotions like guilt or hopelessness about weight loss.

While eating can decrease unwanted emotions, emotions are usually only lessened during eating, not afterward, setting up a cycle that leads to more eating. Let's look at Megan's experience to see how this cycle works. Worry about college or an upcoming test triggers Megan's emotional eating, and as she eats, her anxiety decreases. When she stops eating, her anxiety returns, often accompanied by guilt and hopelessness about losing weight, which triggers more eating.

Does this cycle look familiar? To fully understand the cycle, let's examine how eating decreases emotions. There are several possible psychological or physiological mechanisms:

- ◆ *Eating as a distraction.* For some people, eating becomes a habitual way to distract themselves from unwanted emotions.

- ◆ *Eating as an attempt to engage the relaxation response.* Eating and digestion are the part of the nervous system that's responsible for the relaxation response, so eating can be a way to try to turn on this part of the nervous system.

- ◆ *Eating as a way to numb emotions.* Some people feel numb while eating (binge eating is the kind of eating most likely to produce numbing). If it's extreme, the emotional numbing produces an altered state of consciousness, sometimes called *dissociation* (sort of like an out-of-body experience), that suppresses emotions.

It's important to understand which mechanism is involved in your emotional eating. Josie sometimes feels numb when she eats. This is particularly true when she eats a large amount of high-carbohydrate, high-fat foods, like chips. We can see this on her baseline food log in chapter 6 when she recorded that she felt nothing when bingeing. For Mark it's often about distraction. When Mark is upset, he habitually distracts himself with food. Megan goes for the relaxation response. Answer the following questions about your emotional eating.

Emotional Eating Mechanism Questionnaire

Check the statements in each column that are true for you.

☐ When I eat, I forget about what's bothering me, but I don't feel numb. ☐ I eat when I'm bored. ☐ When I eat, I think of things other than what's bothering me.	☐ I often eat when I'm anxious or worried. ☐ Eating helps me feel more relaxed. ☐ If I eat when I'm nervous, I sometimes get sleepy.	☐ Sometimes I feel numb while eating. ☐ Sometimes I have a sort of out-of-body experience when I eat. ☐ I sometimes lose track of time and what's going on around me when I eat.
Distraction If you checked off any statements above, you may be using emotional eating to distract yourself from difficult emotions.	**Relaxation Response** If you checked off any statements in this column, you may be eating to trigger the relaxation response.	**Emotional Numbing** If you checked off any statements above, you may be triggering an altered state of consciousness that suppresses difficult emotions.

Which statements did you check? While it's possible to use all three emotional eating mechanisms, most people find that they use one mechanism more often than the other two: *The emotional eating mechanism I use the most is:* _____.

Boredom and Eating

Do you eat when you're bored? Eating out of boredom is a common habit. Change your boredom-eating habit by substituting nonfood activities for eating. Keep track of eating out of boredom on your self-monitoring food log. Once you develop awareness of the boredom trigger, substitute other activities for eating. Try calling a friend, working on a hobby, taking a walk, or reading a book.

IDENTIFYING EMOTIONAL EATING

To eliminate emotional eating, you first need to identify your emotional eating habits. It shouldn't surprise you that identifying emotional eating involves collecting data. Use the "Emotions" column on your self-monitoring food log to collect data about emotional eating. Let's look at part of Mark's log to see how this works.

Mark's Self-Monitoring Food Log Day: __7/10/10__ (day before wedding anniversary)

Schedule	Food/Amount	Ate Mindfully	Problem Eating	Emotions	Adhered to Plan/Solutions
☑ Meal ☐ Snack ☐ Unplanned eating Time: Noon	Two fast-food burgers with double meat, a large pack of fries, and soda	☐ Yes ☑ No	Binge	Before: Angry/sad During: Felt better, less angry After: Defeated	☐ Yes ☑ No If no, what happened? My lunch was in the refrigerator, but I felt down and angry about my wedding anniversary tomorrow. Trying to avoid thinking about my divorce led me to get the fast-food take-out. While I was driving to get the food and eating, I sort of forgot about my anniversary.

Next day (Mark's anniversary)

Schedule	Food/Amount	Ate Mindfully	Problem Eating	Emotions	Adhered to Plan/Solutions
☐ Meal ☐ Snack ☑ Unplanned eating Time: 10:00 p.m.	Four pieces of toast with lots of butter and jam	☐ Yes ☑ No		Before: Agitated/hopeless During: Relaxed After: Tired	☐ Yes ☑ No If no, what happened? My daughter called. We talked about her mother. Got off the phone, couldn't relax; knew I wouldn't be able to sleep. Made toast. Went to bed.

Looking at Mark's log, we can see that:

1. Mark was experiencing anger and sadness the day he binged on fast food and experiencing agitation and hopelessness the next day, when he ate the toast.

2. He marked both eating episodes as not mindful. Emotional eating is rarely mindful.

3. He ate high-carbohydrate, high-fat foods, which are common emotional eating foods. As with binge eating, emotional eating rarely involves leafy greens!

4. Eating was unplanned on day two. Emotional eating is often unplanned.

5. He experienced an *emotional vulnerability*, which is something that makes strong emotions more likely. Mark's anniversary was an emotional vulnerability.

6. Mark was distracting himself from his emotions on day one, which included driving to a fast-food restaurant and ordering food. Some people start to feel better while preparing to eat. On the second day, the toast may have been a distraction, but it's also likely Mark was trying to trigger the relaxation response by eating in order to get to sleep.

Emotional Eating Clues

When you review your eating, look for these emotional eating clues:

- Intense unwanted emotions
- High-carbohydrate, high-fat foods
- Emotional vulnerability

- Lack of mindfulness
- Unplanned eating
- Binge eating

Look over your self-monitoring food logs for times you think you engaged in emotional eating. How many episodes of emotional eating do you find? Next, write a description of two episodes of emotional eating:

	What happened?	Emotions before eating	Emotions while eating	Emotions after eating	Did emotions after eating lead to more eating?
1.					☐ Yes ☐ No
2.					☐ Yes ☐ No

EMOTIONAL EATING SOLUTIONS

Now that you've had some experience identifying your emotional eating habits, it's time to look at solutions. We'll start with emotional eating that's meant to distract you from difficult emotions.

Distraction

Distracting yourself from strong unwanted emotions can be a healthy way to cope. What if Mark had distracted himself with something other than food? He drove to get fast food; he could just as easily have driven to the gym for an extra workout or gone to a movie or to visit his grandchildren. There are lots of ways to distract yourself temporarily from difficult emotions. From the following list, check things you can do to distract yourself, and add at least two ideas of your own:

- ☐ Read.
- ☐ Watch a movie.
- ☐ Exercise.
- ☐ Garden.
- ☐ Take your dog for a walk.
- ☐ Do a household chore.
- ☐ Call a friend.
- ☐ Other: _____
- ☐ Other: _____

Relaxation Response

Self-soothing behaviors are activities that lead to relaxation. Self-soothing can be anything from taking a warm bath to listening to soft music. Check which soothing activities you plan to use, and add at least two of your own:

- ☐ Take a warm bath or shower.
- ☐ Listen to soothing music.
- ☐ Watch birds or fish.
- ☐ Pet a dog, cat, or other animal.
- ☐ Knit.

☐ Take a stroll.

☐ Other: _____

☐ Other: _____

Triggering deep relaxation requires more than soothing. Meditation, yoga, and even prayer can trigger a deep relaxation response. Consider taking a meditation or yoga class (we're talking about the gentle forms of yoga; no headstands necessary). Triggering the relaxation response is about practice. Most people find that spending time each day practicing the relaxation response decreases stress and anxiety all day.

Waves of Emotion

Emotions come in waves. At the peak of an unwanted emotion, you may feel as if the emotion will never go away, but the truth is that even very strong emotions like panic or extreme sadness dissipate over time, like how a wave hits the beach. This means that postponing eating when you feel strong unwanted emotions can prevent emotional eating. Every time you experience the peak of a strong emotion without food, it'll be easier to avoid eating when the next wave of emotion hits. Try using distraction or self-soothing until the strength of the emotion decreases, and remind yourself that emotions, like waves, dissipate over time.

Emotional Numbing

The first strategy for combating emotional numbing is *not* eating when you're experiencing strong unwanted emotions. If a strong emotion occurs when it's time to eat, this is the one time you'll need to postpone eating. Take care of yourself by distracting or practicing self-soothing. After the emotion diminishes, eat your scheduled meal or snack. Eat mindfully by noticing the taste, texture, and smell of your food. Slow down and focus on eating.

If you think you're dissociating while eating, consider the possibility that you have a psychological disorder that needs treatment before WLS. People with binge-eating disorder, and those with serious symptoms of depression or anxiety, sometimes dissociate while eating. We'll discuss what to do if you think you have a depressive or anxiety disorder or an eating disorder at the end of this chapter.

PRACTICING SOLUTIONS TO EMOTIONAL EATING

Before you work out your emotional eating solutions, review Mark's solution for the fast-food binge he experienced the day before his wedding anniversary.

Mark's Example	
Mark's Solution	*To make Mark's solution work, he would have needed to...*
I love to drive and always feel more relaxed while driving. I could have taken a drive into the hills around my house.	*I would've needed to take my lunch with me on the drive. It was all prepared; if I didn't take it, I would've gotten too hungry and might have gone through the fast-food lane anyway.*

Review the two episodes of emotional eating you just documented. Put yourself back in the situation in your mind. If you hadn't eaten, what could you have done instead? What would you have needed to do to make your solution work? Next, fill out the solutions for your emotional eating:

My Examples	
My Solution	*To make my solution work, I would have needed to...*
Example 1:	
Example 2:	

TAKING CARE OF DEPRESSION AND ANXIETY SYMPTOMS

Many obese people experience sadness or anxiety about being obese. Obesity also increases your risk of experiencing a depressive or anxiety disorder (Norris 2007). While dysphoria or anxiety that's tied to weight usually resolves with weight loss, if you have a true psychological disorder, like major depressive disorder or generalized anxiety disorder, your symptoms of depression or anxiety will probably persist after weight loss. Answer the following screening questions about how you've felt over the past two to four weeks to see if you are experiencing signs of a depressive or anxiety disorder.

Depressive Disorder/Anxiety Disorder Screen		
Depression		
Do you feel down, sad, or depressed most of the time?	Yes	No
Have you lost interest in activities you used to enjoy?	Yes	No
Do you feel more down in the morning than at other times of day?	Yes	No
Do you feel hopeless or think about dying?	Yes	No
Anxiety		
Do you ruminate about things other than food or weight?	Yes	No
Does worry interfere with your sleep?	Yes	No
Do you sometimes feel so panicky that you avoid doing normal, routine things like driving on the freeway or going to the mall?	Yes	No
Do you wash your hands over and over again, or check and recheck doors, locks, and appliances many times?	Yes	No

Did you answer yes to any of the screening questions? If you answered yes to more than one depression or anxiety question, or to the question about feeling hopeless and thinking about dying, see a mental health professional for an evaluation. It's important to remember that these are only screening questions. A yes answer to any of these questions doesn't necessarily mean you have a depressive or anxiety disorder. Only an evaluation by a mental health professional can determine whether you have a psychological disorder. If you do have a depressive or anxiety disorder, your symptoms should be well controlled or in remission before WLS. Most such disorders are responsive to cognitive behavioral therapy (CBT). If you still have symptoms after CBT treatment, consider talking to your doctor about adding medication.

EATING DISORDERS

If you've been self-monitoring and doing the activities in this chapter and the three previous ones and you're still binge eating more than once a month, doing any purging, or eating at night and not remembering eating, it's time to see an eating-disorder specialist for help. Don't wait; an untreated eating disorder can postpone your surgery and will lead to inadequate weight loss or weight regain.

WHAT'S NEXT?

The lifestyle changes you need to make to prepare for and be successful after WLS are easier if you have good social support. In the next chapter we'll look at mobilizing your social support.

Chapter 10

Mobilizing Your Social Support

If your family and friends don't understand how important it is for you to change your eating habits, it'll be more difficult for you to prepare for WLS and follow the postsurgery lifestyle. In addition to family and friends, others who have had WLS can also provide valuable support. Attending a support group in person or online before and after WLS will give you the opportunity to learn from others. Let's start with mobilizing support from family and friends.

FAMILY AND FRIENDS

There are two basic decisions you need to make about family and friends. The first decision is whom to disclose your WLS plans to. The second decision is what kind of support you want from those close to you.

Whom Do You Plan to Tell?

Mobilizing support doesn't mean you need to tell everyone. You may be comfortable letting most people in your life know, or you may feel more comfortable telling only a few people. Even if you intend to keep your plans mostly private, it's a good idea to talk to a couple of close family members or friends before surgery. Choose people who can give you support during your preparation for WLS and also support you after surgery.

To Tell or Not to Tell

When deciding whom to tell, consider these questions:

1. Are you an open person who is usually comfortable sharing personal information?
   ☐ Yes ☐ No

2. In your family, are family members expected to share most important decisions?
   ☐ Yes ☐ No

3. Are there people in your life who'll notice and ask you about changes in your food choices?
   ☐ Yes ☐ No

4. Is there anyone in your life who has been critical of your weight?   ☐ Yes ☐ No

5. Is there anyone you plan to tell only after surgery, not before?   ☐ Yes ☐ No

6. Do you know someone who has had WLS surgery?   ☐ Yes ☐ No

7. How hard do you think it will be to keep your plans for WLS to yourself?
   ☐ Easy   ☐ Somewhat difficult   ☐ Very difficult

8. Are there any other factors you think are important in deciding whom to tell?

   _____

   _____

Recall how you answered the questions in the previous box while we look at Josie's answers:

1. She's naturally open with friends, family, and coworkers.

2. Her family is the kind of family that shares a lot.

3. Her Friday-night-dinner friends will probably notice that she's eating differently and ask her about it.

4. There's no one she's close to who's negative about her weight.

5. There isn't anyone whom she feels she should wait until after surgery to tell.

6. There's no one she's close to who has had WLS.

7. Josie thinks it will be hard to keep her decision to herself.

Consistent with her answers, after talking with her sisters and aunt, the first people Josie talks to about her surgery are the group of friends she meets on Fridays for dinner. Josie is pleasantly surprised to find that another person in the group is also considering WLS. In contrast to Josie, Mark rarely eats meals with anyone other than his daughters and their families, so he decides to tell his adult daughters and one close friend who is post-WLS. Mark thinks he can get useful support from his friend, who is doing well with weight-loss maintenance. Mark chooses not to tell his brother, Jim, whom he sees only a few times a year. Jim's past comments about Mark's needing to "Just stop eating" lead Mark to believe it's better to tell his brother after surgery, when his weight loss is evident. In this space below, write the names of the people you plan to confide in before surgery. Next to each name, write why you're choosing to tell that person:

Name: _____ Why: _____

Name: _____ Why: _____

Name: _____ Why: _____

List the names of anyone in your life you plan to tell after surgery and why you're waiting:

Name: _____ Why: _____

Name: _____ Why: _____

When You Don't Want to Tell

WLS is a personal medical decision, but it's one that can be hard to keep completely to yourself. Sometimes the choice to keep WLS confidential is based in a sense of privacy, but other times, the reason to keep quiet about surgery is *unjustified shame*. Unjustified shame is shame that's based on faulty reasoning, a common example being *I should be able to lose weight and keep the weight off on my own, without surgery*. This faulty reasoning is in direct contrast to what we learned in chapter 1. The fact is that getting healthy requires tools, and WLS is a tool that's more effective than conventional diet and exercise for morbidly obese people, *and* surgically assisted weight loss still requires work. There's no shame in carefully choosing an effective tool and committing yourself to the work required to make the tool work for you.

Once you have surgery and lose weight, it can be even harder to keep your surgery confidential. Ask yourself:

◆ *Am I a private person who likes to keep personal things like WLS confidential?*

◆ *Do I want confidentiality because I'm ashamed I couldn't lose weight without surgery?*

If you're a private person who doesn't want to answer every question about your eating habits or weight with a WLS discussion, or if there's someone you definitely don't want to tell, you need to find a neutral answer to questions like "Why aren't you eating the rice?" "Wow, you've lost a lot of weight! What's your secret?" or "Did you do something to lose weight?" Try these neutral answers:

- "Just working on being healthier."

- "I'm just not hungry."

- "I'm following a healthier eating plan."

With the increase in WLS prevalence, some people assume that significant weight loss equals WLS, so you may get a direct question. If you're a private person, you'll have to decide whether you will:

- Change the subject.

- Tell your inquisitor this is a private question you won't answer.

- Lie.

On the other hand, if your reluctance to tell is based in shame, to rid yourself of shame, try to:

- Acknowledge to yourself that your shame is unjustified. There's no shame in taking action to improve your health.

- Reread the information in chapter 1 to better understand the effectiveness of the WLS tool.

- Join a support group and talk to others who've had WLS.

- Start telling people. A good way to get rid of unjustified shame is to do what makes you feel shameful.

What Kind of Support Do You Want?

There are different kinds of support people can give you. Next, check the kinds of support you think you need. From your previous list, add the person (or people) who will provide that support:

☐ Someone to act as a sounding board to help you process all the WLS information. Who: _____

☐ An exercise buddy. Who: _____

☐ Someone to support you in changing the way you eat as you prepare for WLS. This can mean a family member who's willing to get rid of all the junk food in the house or a coworker who will brown-bag it with you instead of going out for fast food. Who: _____

☐ Someone to attend doctor's appointments with you. Who: _____

☐ Someone to help you at the time of your surgery. You'll need someone to drive you home, and you may need someone to stay with you for a few days after surgery. Who: _____

☐ Someone to care for children or pets while you are in the hospital.

Who: _____

☐ Other support you think you'll need: _____

Who: _____

Now that you've identified your support team, it's time to educate them. While some members of your support team might need to know only the kind of food your cat likes so your cat can stay fed while you are in the hospital, most members of your support team will need to know more. It's always a good idea to educate people you cook for, eat with, or live with. Anyone in your life (like a spouse or partner) who needs a comprehensive understanding of the risks and benefits of WLS will benefit from reading the first part of this book.

What If Someone in Your Life Objects to Your Having WLS?

You might find that someone in your life doesn't think WLS is a good idea. Often the objection comes from fear about the surgery, but sometimes it stems from a philosophical belief that WLS is somehow the easy way out. If the objections come from someone important to you, it's a good idea to set up a time to talk about WLS. Review these tips to help you make the conversation productive:

1. Listen carefully to what the person says to learn what the objection is. Don't interrupt; let the person explain his objections fully before you talk.

2. Thank the person for explaining his objections and for agreeing to talk.

3. If the objections are anxiety based (for example, perhaps the person has heard that people can die during surgery), ask if he's willing to learn more about WLS risks. Without minimizing the surgery risks, explain that the risks to your health are serious if you don't lose weight. If the person is very close to you, consider:

   ◆ Sharing the information about WLS complications

   ◆ Inviting the person to go with you to your appointment with the surgeon

   ◆ Sharing the resources section in the back of the book

4. Be patient! Keep in mind that if the person didn't care about you, he wouldn't be so worried.

5. If the objection is more philosophical, take some time to explain your position, and let the person know that WLS is a tool, not an easy way out. When the person hears how much you'll have to change your eating habits and lifestyle to make WLS successful, he may realize that WLS is not easy. In the end, if your loved one feels strongly about his position, you might have to agree to disagree. Seek support from others in your life as you prepare for WLS.

SUPPORT GROUPS FOR WLS

Attending a WLS support group can help you lose weight after surgery (Song et al. 2008). In addition to leading to better weight loss, attending a support group can help you prepare for surgery, which is why some WLS programs require that you attend a support group before surgery.

Support groups differ depending on who facilitates the group. You can find professionally facilitated groups at many WLS centers that often focus on education as well as support. Self-help support groups are usually facilitated by someone who has had WLS. Visiting a few support groups, perhaps one of each type, is a good way to find the right fit. To find support groups in your area, call your local WLS center, or go online and search for "WLS support." There are several national listings of WLS support groups (see the resources section in the back of the book). Online support groups are growing in popularity. They give you the opportunity to talk with people from all over the United States or, sometimes, around the world.

WHAT'S NEXT?

Bariatric surgery requires a team. In the next chapter we'll discuss key members of the WLS team and what you can expect when you meet with each team member.

Chapter 11

Meeting with Your Weight Loss Surgery Team

In this chapter you'll learn what to expect when you meet with your surgeon and the psychologist who does your psychological evaluation. Registered dietitians are important members of any WLS team, so we'll explore the information you can expect from your appointment with the dietitian. We'll also discuss presurgery orientation classes, diets, and roadblocks. Roadblocks include wanting a different WLS than the one your surgeon recommends, experiencing an insurance denial, or not being cleared for surgery by the psychologist.

YOUR TEAM

You'll come in contact with many medical professionals during your presurgery appointments and surgery. Before surgery, part of your job is to show these medical professionals that you are prepared for WLS and understand the significant lifestyle changes WLS requires. Appointments with these three types of medical professionals will be particularly important in determining your readiness for surgery and what type of WLS is most appropriate for you:

- Surgeon
- Psychologist
- Registered dietitian

In addition to attending appointments with these professionals, you may be asked to attend an orientation class. Whether or not you're required to attend classes will depend on the requirements of your WLS program. Large WLS programs tend to require more in the way of education than private-practice surgeons do. Let's look at what happens in an orientation and then examine in detail what you can expect from appointments with the surgeon, psychologist, and dietitian.

Orientation

It's possible that your first WLS appointment will be an orientation class. The orientation is your opportunity to ask questions and find out about specific requirements of the WLS program. Take a notebook, so you can take notes and be prepared to ask questions. Here are some suggested questions:

- *What types of WLS does the program perform?*

- *Will I have to lose weight before surgery?*

- *What support does the program provide after surgery?*

- *How many surgeries do the program or surgeons perform each year?*

- *What insurance coverage does the program accept?*

Surgeon

Meeting with a surgeon is an exciting step in the process. Depending on your WLS program, you may meet with your surgeon right away, after seeing the psychologist and dietitian, or after attending the orientation. If you're planning to have your surgery in a large WLS program, you can expect the program to do at least two types of surgeries. If you go to a smaller private practice, you may find that the surgeon does only one type of WLS (usually gastric banding), so make sure you ask what kind of WLS the surgeon performs. Don't assume you'll remember all the questions you want to ask; take a list with you. It's helpful to review the information in chapter 2 before your appointment, so you can ask questions about complications and different types of WLS. Here are some questions to consider asking:

- *Which types of WLS do you perform?*

- *How many surgeries have you performed?*

- *Given my weight and medical conditions, which WLS do you think is most appropriate for me?*

- *How much of my excess weight can I expect to lose with the type of surgery you recommend?* (This is a very important question to ask, because the surgeon's response will help you determine your weight loss goal.)

- *What medical tests will I have before WLS?*

- *Given my overall health, what complications should I worry about?*

- *What vitamins do you recommend after WLS?*

- *What regular lab tests should I have after WLS?*

- *How much loose skin do you think I'll have?*

- *How long will I stay in the hospital?*

- *How long will I be off work?*

Why Is My Surgeon Asking Me to Lose Weight Before Surgery?

While not all surgeons ask patients to diet and lose weight before surgery, many do. Losing weight before surgery removes fat from your liver. Fat in the liver increases the chances of surgical complications. In addition even a 10 percent weight loss can help you get diabetes and other chronic medical conditions under better control before surgery (Kurian, Thompson, and Davidson 2005). If you do need to diet before surgery, be sure to ask the surgeon how much weight you need to lose.

Psychologist

A psychologist will evaluate you for psychological appropriateness and WLS readiness. If the WLS program you are participating in doesn't have a staff psychologist, ask for a referral to a psychologist who has experience in doing WLS evaluations. The purpose of the psychological evaluation, which is usually completed in one or two appointments, is to answer these questions:

- Do you have a psychological disorder that would interfere with your ability to adapt to the lifestyle changes WLS requires?

- Do you have a psychological disorder (including an eating disorder) that should be treated before surgery?

- Are you engaging in emotional eating?

- Do you have social support to help you after WLS?

- Are you preparing for surgery by changing your eating habits?

- Are you prepared to lose weight before surgery if your surgeon requires it?

- Do you have realistic expectations for how WLS will change your body and life?

- Do you have a realistic expectation of how much weight you will lose?

- Are you prepared to deal with WLS aftereffects like loose skin?

- How do you think about food?

◆ Do you smoke tobacco, use drugs, or drink alcohol?

In addition to an interview, most psychologists administer psychological testing as part of the evaluation. These are usually paper-and-pencil tests (inkblots don't apply) that normally include assessment of symptoms of a possible psychological disorder, evaluation of your thinking about food and weight, and evaluation of your quality of life. The psychologist should explain the purpose of each test. If you don't understand the purpose of the test or its instructions, say so. Don't complete a psychological test if you don't understand why you're taking it. Some psychologists also look at food logs as part of the evaluation, so it's a good idea to bring your food logs to the appointment. While some psychologists may ask you a few questions about your childhood, a difficult childhood or a history of childhood abuse shouldn't prevent you from having WLS. Studies of patients who've experienced abuse find that a history of abuse doesn't affect WLS outcomes, so many psychologists who specialize in WLS consider this kind of information irrelevant unless you're experiencing current symptoms of a psychological disorder connected to the abuse (Grilo et al. 2006). If you're currently in an abusive relationship, this *is* relevant because it could affect your ability to cope after WLS. Psychologists usually also evaluate for tobacco, drug, or alcohol use. Smoking increases your chances of surgical complications. If you smoke, you'll need to stop before surgery. Most surgeons won't perform surgery on someone who smokes. If you're abusing alcohol or drugs, you'll need to be clean and sober for a period of time before surgery. Finally, if you've been in treatment for an eating disorder or some other psychological disorder in the past two years, you may need to get a letter from your treating mental health provider that indicates your symptoms are under control or in remission.

Dietitian

You'll have at least one appointment with a registered dietitian. Dietitians are good sources of information on how to eat after WLS, and they sometimes offer nutritional classes for people seeking WLS. If your WLS program provides these classes, it's a good idea to attend. The more information you have, the better prepared you will be. At some point before surgery, a dietitian will evaluate your eating, usually by reviewing your food logs. As with the surgeon and psychologist, it's a good idea to go to your appointment with a list of written questions. Questions to ask the dietitian include:

◆ *How much protein should I eat every day after WLS?*

◆ *What are good sources of lean protein?*

◆ *Can you review my food log and tell me how I can improve my eating so that I'll be ready for WLS?*

If your religion requires dietary restrictions or you're a vegetarian, talk to the dietitian about post-surgery eating, given your restrictions.

DEALING WITH BARRIERS

At this point in your preparation for WLS, three barriers can occur: the surgeon could recommend a type of WLS you don't want, your insurance company could deny coverage for WLS or for the type of surgery your surgeon recommends, or the psychologist could tell you you're not ready for surgery. Let's look at these possible barriers and how to deal with each.

What to Do If the Surgeon Recommends a Different WLS

It's possible the surgeon will recommend a different type of WLS than you want. If this happens, the first thing to do is to ask the surgeon why she's suggesting the type of surgery she recommends. Listen carefully to her reasons. If you still want to pursue a different surgery after listening to all the medical reasons for the one recommended, seek a second opinion from a different surgeon. If the second surgeon recommends the same surgery as the first, it's time to rethink your choice of surgery.

What to Do If Your Insurance Denies Coverage of Your WLS

It's possible to run into barriers with your health insurance company. Two insurance barriers can occur: your insurance carrier can refuse to cover the type of WLS the surgeon recommends or deny coverage for any type of WLS. Make sure you're familiar with the details of your policy. While filling out paperwork can be frustrating, it's important to make sure you have completed all the required forms. Ask for a letter of medical necessity from the surgeon that explains medically why you need WLS, so you can submit it to your insurance company. If you don't meet the NIH guidelines for WLS discussed in chapter 1, it may be difficult for you to get your insurance company to cover your surgery. If you're not approved, find out what the appeal process is. Don't give up; if you're persistent and can document medical necessity for WLS, you may be successful with your appeal.

What to Do If the Psychologist Thinks You're Not Ready for WLS

After your evaluation with the psychologist, if she tells you she thinks you're not ready for surgery, don't panic. Make sure you ask exactly why she thinks you're not ready. Common reasons people aren't ready for WLS include:

◆ You haven't resolved eating problems or have an eating disorder that's not in remission.

- You have current symptoms of a psychological disorder, like major depressive disorder, that requires treatment before WLS.

- You're not prepared to change your eating habits after WLS.

- You have unrealistic ideas about what WLS will do for you.

When you have a good understanding of why the psychologist feels you aren't ready, ask her what you can do to improve your readiness for surgery. There's almost always something you can do. Ask when you can repeat the psychological evaluation, and work on resolving the issues the psychologist is concerned about.

WHAT'S NEXT?

You have put a lot of work into getting ready for WLS. As the day of your surgery gets closer, you may find yourself feeling fear and excitement at the same time. In the next chapter we'll discuss what to expect from surgery, including what to expect during your hospital stay and what to expect the first week or two after your surgery.

Chapter 12

Undergoing Surgery

In this chapter we'll discuss what to expect during your hospital stay, plus what to expect in the first days and weeks after WLS. Having a realistic weight-loss goal is important. Without a goal it's harder to feel as if you're making progress in your weight-loss journey. By the end of this chapter, you'll have a realistic weight-loss goal so you can start tracking your weight loss as soon as you leave the hospital. You've put in a lot of effort preparing for surgery, but in many ways your journey has just begun. Let's start with your hospital stay.

HOSPITAL STAY

Unless you experience surgical complications, you can expect your hospital stay to be short. Today few surgeries require more than a few days in the hospital, and WLS is no exception. The length of your hospital stay depends on a number of factors, including:

- The type of WLS

- Your overall health

- How much support you have at home

It's not just the length of the hospital stay that has changed; the days of patients lying in bed after surgery are long gone. Within hours of surgery, you'll probably be asked to stand and take a few steps. If you've been diligent about following your exercise plan, getting up will be much easier for you.

It may be helpful to have someone stay with you while you are in the hospital. Some hospitals allow a family member to be with you overnight. Make sure you know hospital rules about visitors ahead of time. Review this hospital-stay checklist:

☐ Ask about rules for visitors.

☐ Arrange for someone to take you home after WLS; you won't be able to drive yourself right away.

☐ Depending on the WLS you have and your overall health, you may want to have someone stay with you for a few days after surgery. If you live alone, ask your surgeon if he thinks you need someone to stay with you for a day or two.

☐ If you have small children, arrange for someone to help you with the kids for a few days. You won't be able to lift and carry your child when you first get home. Someone who can help you by picking up your crying toddler when you can't will make the first few days less stressful on everyone.

☐ Before your surgery, purchase enough postsurgery vitamins and food for the first couple of weeks after surgery. You'll start taking vitamins right away.

WHAT TO EXPECT IN THE FIRST FEW WEEKS

Before surgery your surgeon or registered dietitian will give you a specific diet to follow after surgery. You'll probably have an appointment with your dietitian a week or two after your surgery. The postsurgery diet is usually presented in stages, with guidelines at each stage for moving on to the next stage. As with most surgeries, you'll start out with clear liquids (stage 1) and slowly move toward solid food as you recover. Recommendations differ depending on which WLS you have and how well you're doing. Carefully follow the instructions you're given. Here are the typical stages of the post-WLS diet (Aills et al. 2008):

- ◆ *Stage 1* (Day after WLS) Clear liquid diet: (for example, high-protein broth)

- ◆ *Stage 2:* Full liquid diet (for example, protein shakes), possibly starting as early as the day after surgery

- ◆ *Stage 3:* Pureed/soft diet (for example, scrambled eggs); stage 3 usually lasts about two weeks

- ◆ *Stage 4:* Soft foods (for example, finely ground tuna); some WLS recommendations combine stages 3 and 4

- ◆ *Post-WLS diet:* Eating for the rest of your life

Important: These are general guidelines depending on your health. If anything here contradicts your surgeon's recommendations, follow your surgeon's recommendations rather than these guidelines.

POSTSURGERY PROBLEMS: WHEN TO CALL YOUR DOCTOR

Feeling tired and even a little weak after surgery is normal. Surgery is an assault on your body, and you can't expect to feel great in the week or so afterward. Occasionally surgical complications occur after leaving the hospital. If you experience any of these symptoms, call your surgeon (Kurian, Thompson, and Davidson 2005):

◆ Excessive bleeding, swelling, or drainage from your incision

◆ Excessive redness around your incision

◆ Unusual pain in your lower extremities

◆ Shoulder pain

◆ Body temperature above 100 degrees Fahrenheit (37.7 degrees Celsius)

◆ Shaking or chills, increased fatigue, or shortness of breath

◆ Worsening abdominal pain

◆ Inability to eat or drink

◆ Excessive vomiting or nausea

◆ Fainting

◆ Black stools or blood in your stools

◆ Very dark urine or inability to urinate

◆ Diarrhea that's pure water

◆ Other signs your surgeon told you to watch for

RETURNING TO WORK

Your surgeon will let you know when you can return to work. The type of surgery you have, your age, how well your recovery is going, and the kind of work you do are all factors in determining when it's safe for you to return to work. Finding out from your employer whether your work can be modified may allow you to return to work sooner. If you normally do physical work but your employer can assign you less physical work for a few days or weeks, your surgeon may let you return with restrictions or allow you to return part-time so you don't get too tired. Restrictions mean you can do some kinds of work but not others. Lifting is one of the work duties you probably won't be able to perform right away, so if you work in a warehouse and your employer can't accommodate your lifting restrictions, expect to be out for a longer period of time.

If you haven't told your coworkers about your surgery, before you return to work, decide what you're comfortable telling people. Review chapter 10 if you're not sure whom to tell. If you work at a company with a hundred or more people, someone else at your company has probably also had WLS. Obesity-related lost workdays have become common enough that some large companies have weight control or even WLS support groups on-site. Several of my patients received support from management to start WLS support groups at work. Sitting together at lunch with others who've had WLS or coworkers who are working on losing weight with conventional dieting can be a lot more fun than sitting with people who don't understand why you're passing up the lunch truck's offerings.

SELF-MONITORING

You may have thought that now that you've had surgery, you can forget about self-monitoring. The truth is keeping a log is as important after WLS as it was before. Keeping your self-monitoring food log after WLS can help you:

- ◆ Ensure that you're eating enough protein
- ◆ Discover which foods don't agree with your new digestive system
- ◆ Lose weight
- ◆ Stop or prevent weight regain

Use the following log for your post-WLS monitoring, or if you have been using an electronic log, you can continue to use your electronic log as long as it allows you to track protein grams. The last column of the log, "Observations or Changes I Need to Make," is intended to help you correct your course if you get off track. Say you skip breakfast. Note that in this column and write what you need to do to correct the problem. If you find that certain situations, like social events, are a problem, make a note of that observation and write your ideas for dealing with the next social event. As with the other logs, the point is to make the log a tool that works for you, so add anything to the log you think might help you. At the bottom of the log is a place to document your exercise for the day, including how much time you spent exercising and a section for your weight. Particularly in the beginning, you might want to weigh yourself daily. In the first few months after surgery, you may see a daily change in your weight.

Post-WLS Self-Monitoring Food Log   Day: _____

Time and Location	Food/Drink	Amount	Protein grams	Observations or Changes I Need to Make
Breakfast:				
Lunch:				
Dinner				
Additional:				
Exercise:	Time:			
Weight Today:				

WEIGHT LOSS GOAL

It's important to have a weight loss goal to work toward. Consider the goal you form now to be a working goal, meaning you may need to change it as time goes on. One of the common weight-loss patterns is hitting a low weight and regaining a few pounds before your weight stabilizes. Possibly related to changes in metabolism and absorption, this pattern isn't usually a problem unless your weight continues to increase. We'll talk more about this pattern in chapter 16.

In chapter 1 we learned that it's common to have unrealistic expectations for weight loss after WLS. You may recall that depending on your type of weight loss surgery, you can expect to lose 40 to 70 percent of your excess weight, with gastric banding producing the least amount of weight loss (Tice et al. 2008). While it might seem disappointing to expect to lose less than 100 percent of your excess weight, a 40 to 70 percent weight loss is far above what conventional diet and exercise produce. In chapter 1 you calculated your excess weight by determining the amount of weight you needed to lose to be in the middle of the normal BMI range. Then you calculated how much weight you'd need to lose for a weight loss of 40 to 70 percent of your excess weight. You probably also had a discussion with your surgeon before surgery about how much weight you could expect to lose with your type of surgery. Review your calculations in chapter 1 and combine that information with what your surgeon told you. What do you think is a reasonable weight goal based on your excess weight and the information from your surgeon? Next, write the goal and the number of pounds you need to lose to reach that goal.

My realistic goal weight is: _____ *pounds.*

Weight loss goal: to reach my goal weight, I need to lose: _____ *pounds.*

When you see your surgeon for your postsurgery follow-up appointment, discuss your weight goal with him. Ask him if he thinks you're being realistic. Adjust your goal based on your surgeon's feedback and write the goal and the pounds you need to lose to make that goal at the top of the weight loss chart at the end of this chapter.

Once you've reached your goal weight, your new goal will be to keep your weight stable. It's normal for your body weight to fluctuate within a five-pound range. Next, calculate your five-pound range by adding and subtracting two and one half pounds to and from your goal weight so that your goal weight is in the middle of the range. This is the range you'll want to stay within.

Five-pound range: _____ *to* _____ .

TRACKING WEIGHT LOSS

Tracking your weight loss is a fun post-WLS task. Track your weight loss on a chart at least once a week, so you can see your weekly weight-loss trend. The greatest weight loss usually occurs in the first six to eight months after surgery, with weight loss slowing or stopping after the first year. If you have a lot of weight to lose, you may keep losing after the first eight months, and if you started your WLS journey in the superobese-BMI range, expect to continue to lose weight into the second year after surgery. In addition to noting your daily weight on your self-monitoring food log, use the pounds-lost chart at the end of this chapter to keep track of your success.

Chart Instructions: Write your goal weight, weight-loss goal (the pounds you need to lose to reach your goal weight), and five-pound range at the top of the chart. At the bottom of the chart, you'll see "Weeks." Along the left side is "Pounds." For each week for the next six months, color in the length of the row of boxes corresponding to the number of pounds you lost that week. The chart will give you a picture of pounds lost over time.

Megan loses seventeen pounds in the first three weeks. Review a sample of Megan's chart to see how she fills in this information.

Pounds	Megan's Weekly Pounds-Lost Chart		
17			
16			
15			
14			
13			
12			
11			
10			
9			
8			
7			
6			
5			
4			
3			
2			
1			
Week —>	1 Lost eight pounds	2 Lost five pounds	3 Lost four pounds

WHAT'S NEXT?

WLS has given you a digestive system that doesn't work like the digestive system you were born with. Now it's time to move on to part 3 and learn how to live successfully with your altered digestive system. While your weight loss will slow as time passes, if your weight loss stops before you reach 50 percent (40 percent if you had gastric banding) of your excess weight, warning bells should go off in your head. In part 3 we'll discuss how to stay on track with eating after surgery. If the pounds aren't coming off, you're probably slipping into old eating habits. If this happens to you, read chapter 13 very carefully, so you can take action right away to continue losing the weight you need to lose.

Goal Weight: _____. Weight Loss Goal: _____ pounds. Five-Pound Range: _____ to _____.

Weekly Pounds-Lost Chart

Pounds																									
40																									
39																									
38																									
37																									
36																									
35																									
34																									
33																									
32																									
31																									
30																									
29																									
28																									
27																									
26																									
25																									
24																									
23																									
22																									

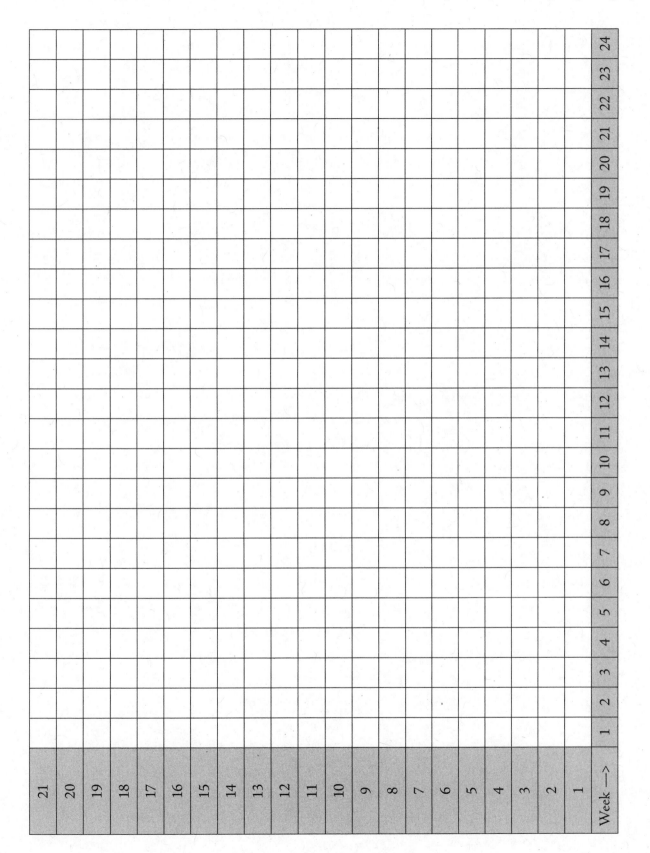

Part 3

Life After Weight Loss Surgery

You've worked hard to reach your goal of having WLS. Now it's time to learn to live your life postsurgery. Life after WLS is not the same as before surgery. Life's not completely different, of course, but it's different in some significant ways. Your willingness to accept the differences is an essential factor in reaching your weight loss goal and living successfully after WLS. We'll start our discussion with what it means to be willing after surgery and how willfulness can sabotage your weight loss and your health. Your digestive system is no longer the normal system you were born with. In the beginning, a post-WLS digestive system doesn't always react to food in a predictable way. It'll take time for you to get to know and understand your new digestive system. In chapter 13 you'll learn what it means to accept and take care of your altered postsurgery digestive system. In chapter 14 we'll look at eating mindfully after WLS, including enjoying food and how to deal with potlucks and other social events. We'll examine body image and coping with post-weight-loss issues like loose skin in chapter 15. Chapter 16 is devoted to avoiding or reversing weight regain. In chapter 17, the last chapter in the book, we'll explore what's next in your life.

Chapter 13

Willingness: Caring for Your Postsurgery Digestive System

WLS changes your digestive system. In this chapter we'll explore what it means to be willing to live with and care for your surgically altered digestive system. Without willingness you probably won't lose enough weight, and you could even develop serious digestive problems. We'll start with how willingness and its opposite, willfulness, can help or hurt your adjustment to your postsurgery digestive system.

WILLINGNESS AND WILLFULNESS

We learned about willingness in chapter 4. Just to review, willingness means accepting what's true about your body and life, then acting effectively based on what's true. When applied to WLS, willingness means accepting these post-WLS truths:

◆ Your digestive system has been altered.

◆ Your altered digestive system requires eating by a different set of rules.

◆ Your digestive system is not as efficient at absorbing vitamins as a normal digestive system.

◆ Your digestive system needs plenty of water.

◆ Eating as you did before WLS can cause digestive problems.

◆ Eating as you did before WLS will interfere with weight loss and promote weight regain.

Accepting these truths is not always easy. Let's look at examples of what it means to act effectively given these truths.

Truth	Effective Action
Your digestive system is now incompatible with alcohol	Passing up the champagne at a friend's wedding reception.
Not eating enough protein will lead to hair and muscle loss.	Carefully tracking how much protein you eat every day.
High-fat foods can cause loose stools or gas.	Checking the fat content of the food you eat.
The French bread at your favorite restaurant isn't the best choice to accompany the grilled chicken breast you ordered.	Ordering vegetables as a side instead.
You'll have to take vitamins every day to stay healthy.	Swallowing all your vitamins even when you don't want to.
You need to drink plenty of water in between meals and snacks.	Carry a water bottle with you everywhere.

Willingness is something we practice moment to moment. No one is willing 100 percent of the time. As we learned in chapter 4, the opposite of willingness is willfulness, which means rejecting what's true and refusing to act effectively. Common ways people ignore post-WLS truths and act willfully include:

◆ Not eating enough protein

◆ Drinking alcohol, caffeine, or carbonated beverages

◆ Eating foods that expand in the stomach, like soft breads and rice

◆ Grazing throughout the day rather than eating three meals a day

◆ Not drinking enough water

◆ Not exercising

◆ Not taking daily vitamins

When we experience a major change in our lives, most of us struggle with moments of willfulness. If you're more than a few weeks past your surgery, you've probably already found it hard to stay willing and accept the truths of your altered digestive system 100 percent of the time. Maybe you've struggled to eat enough protein or pass up your favorite rice dish at a potluck. When has it been difficult for you to accept the truths about your altered insides? When have you slipped into willfulness? In the following box, write when you've been willful.

> *I was willful when:*

There's good news and bad news about willfulness: The bad news is that we can slip into willfulness at any time. The good news is that just because we act willfully doesn't mean we have to stay willful. For example, if you start skipping breakfast or engaging in other willful behavior, as soon as you realize you've been willful, you can move over to willingness. Using the breakfast example, moving over to willingness means making sure you eat as much protein as possible at lunch and dinner and doing what you need to do to ensure that you eat breakfast the next day, whether it's getting up earlier or making your breakfast the night before.

Sometimes the consequences of willfulness show up quickly. When this happens, it's easier to recognize that we've been willful. For example, if you're prone to sugar dumping and you eat the cake at your friend's wedding, you'll feel very sick right away, which might make you think twice about being willful the next time you're faced with something sweet.

While sugar dumping can provide quick feedback about willfulness, other post-WLS consequences of willfulness often don't show up right away. Weight regain can occur early but usually doesn't start until the second or third year after surgery. But we know that how you eat during the first two years is related to weight regain. Unfortunately this delay in consequences makes willful eating seem inconsequential. Foods like rice and soft bread can stretch your stomach, but your stomach won't be stretched from just one bit of rice or bread. The problem is that one bit leads to more as willfulness takes over. Repeated willful eating leads to a stomach that's much bigger than your surgeon intended. Josie discovers this the hard way. While she loses weight at first, her weight loss stops at 35 percent of her excess weight and she starts to gain. When she comes to see me to find out why she hasn't lost more weight and is regaining, we look at her food logs and find that Josie is engaging in several willful eating behaviors. One of her willful behaviors is regularly eating foods that could stretch her stomach. As Josie puts it: "It didn't seem like any big deal to eat a little rice or bread, because I was losing weight. Then without really thinking about it, I was eating rice or bread almost every day." Over time, as a result of stretching her stomach, Josie finds she can eat more of everything. Since her thick, dark hair is one of the things she likes best about her appearance, Josie is diligent about eating enough protein. But her larger stomach capacity leads to her slowly adding high-carbohydrate foods to the protein she eats. Josie is able to get back on track but finds it much harder to lose the weight she regained the second time around. The consequences of Josie's willfulness may be delayed, but in the end they are very serious for her.

CARING FOR YOUR ALTERED DIGESTIVE SYSTEM

An important part of being willing after WLS is learning how to take special care of your altered digestive system. In the beginning you and your new digestive system may not always be on the same page. Adjusting to your new insides means following some important, basic post-WLS rules. In addition to getting adequate protein, you'll need to drink enough water to stay hydrated and be careful around food that's incompatible with your altered digestive system. One of the most common complaints after WLS is altered regularity. You've probably been accustomed to a certain digestive rhythm, and WLS has likely changed that rhythm. If you don't take proper care of your post-WLS digestive system, bowel problems, like constipation or loose stools, and stomach problems, like nausea or difficulty swallowing pills, can interfere with your quality of life. Let's explore how to live comfortably with your new digestive system, starting with a discussion about protein.

The Importance of Protein

By now you may be sick of hearing about protein, but it's so important that we need to touch on one more aspect of protein. Before WLS you needed about 50 grams of protein a day, but 60 to 80 grams a day is a common recommendation after WLS (70 percent if you're still losing) (Aills et al. 2008). If you had the duodenal switch, you'll need even more protein (about 90 grams) (ibid.).

Not eating enough protein can result in more than losing your hair. After WLS, while you're losing fat, you can also lose *fat free mass* (FFM). FFM is everything but fat, the nonfat components of your body, such as muscle. Getting enough protein will help to preserve your FFM as you lose fat. If you don't get enough protein, you can expect (ibid.):

◆ Your muscles to waste as you lose FFM

◆ Your hair to fall out

◆ To feel tired and weak

◆ To become anemic

The protein you eat should be lean but *not* dry or fibrous. Some types of protein tend to be more dry or fibrous. For example, beef can be fibrous and dry. If you plan to eat beef, try to buy the most expensive cut of meat you can. Expensive cuts of beef tend to be less fibrous than cheaper cuts. You'll be eating less volume, so you may find spending more money per pound to be a reasonable trade-off because you'll get more meals out of a pound. In general if you can't chew the meat until it feels like fine mush, you'll have problems swallowing.

Hair Loss

About 30 percent of people who have WLS experience hair loss, usually during the time of greatest rate of weight loss (Kurian, Thompson, and Davidson 2005). While we know that protein deficiencies cause hair loss, other reasons for hair loss aren't completely understood. If you experience hair loss, as long as you're getting enough protein, your hair should grow back over time. Sometimes when hair grows back, it's different, so you could go from curly to straight or straight to curly. If your diet is protein deficient, you'll continue to lose hair.

Always eat your protein first. Once you've finished your protein, you can eat a small amount of vegetables, carbohydrates, or low-sugar fruit, but you may have noticed already that after eating your protein, you have little room left for other foods. We'll talk more about nonprotein foods in the next chapter.

Good Sources of Protein:

- Egg (particularly egg whites)

- Lean but not dry meats (chicken, beef, or pork)

- Fish

- Yogurt (particularly Greek style)

- Fat-free cottage cheese

- Nonfat cow's milk

- Soy milk

- Legumes (with cereals or grains)

Never Miss Your Vitamins

Unless you had a gastric band or the gastric sleeve, you'll need to take vitamins for the rest of your life. Follow your surgeon's recommendations carefully. Here are some common supplementation guidelines:

- Multivitamin and mineral supplement

In addition to a multivitamin and mineral supplement, you may be told to take additional:

- Vitamin B_{12} and folate

- Calcium

- Iron

- Fat-soluble vitamins, such as vitamins D, K, and E

Other supplements you may be asked to take are:

- Micronutrients, such as zinc

- Vitamin B complex

AVOID SUGAR DUMPING

If you had RNYGB and you experience sugar dumping, it means you ate something with a high-carbohydrate or high-fat content. The easiest way to deal with sugar dumping is to avoid it. Remember, fruits that are high in sugar, like oranges and pineapples, can cause sugar dumping. Sugar dumping is miserable but not deadly. Not everyone who has RNYGB experiences sugar dumping. If you're not sure whether you are susceptible to sugar dumping, you might be tempted to conduct a "test" to see what happens. There's only one reason to do this test: to see if you can get away with eating high-carbohydrate or fatty foods. Rather than testing, it's best to eat foods that won't cause sugar dumping. If you do experience sugar dumping, go to bed, if you can, and recommit yourself to caring for your altered digestive system by avoiding sugar and fat.

Dealing with Dehydration

You'll absorb less water from your food after WLS, and because you're no longer drinking with your meals, it's easy to become dehydrated. Don't drink within thirty minutes of starting to eat, and wait at least thirty to sixty minutes after you eat before drinking. But not drinking with meals doesn't mean you can skip drinking water. You need to drink at least 64 ounces of water every day (Kurian, Thompson, and Davidson 2005). Water does these important things for your body:

- Flushes toxins from your kidneys and liver
- Regulates your body temperature
- Helps with digestion
- Lubricates joints
- Promotes muscle energy

If you really dislike drinking pure water, you can add sugarless flavors to it or purchase water that's flavored with artificial sweeteners. Carefully read the label of noncarbonated, artificially flavored water to make sure you're not getting unintended additions like caffeine or salt (sodium).

Not So Regular Anymore

If you were accustomed to having regular bowel movements before surgery, it's time to accept that being regular is different after surgery. It takes time to develop a new "normal regularity," and bowel problems like constipation, loose stools, and gas are common postsurgery problems.

CONSTIPATION

Before your surgery, maybe you were used to having a bowel movement every day. After WLS, bowel movements only every two to three days is considered normal (Kurian, Thompson, and Davidson 2005). If you're having a bowel movement more seldom than once a week or your stools are very hard, you're experiencing constipation. Try this:

- Drink more water.

- Eat a high-fiber, low-sugar cereal.

- Take a fiber preparation like Metamucil, Citrucel, or Benefiber (generics: psyllium, methylcellulose, and wheat dextrin, respectively).

Be patient! Your digestive system has gone through a big change, and it may take time and willingness on your part to accept a new definition of what's regular. If you experience constipation that continues after you've tried the previous suggestions, see your doctor.

DIARRHEA AND LOOSE STOOLS

Lose stools are common after RNYGB and the duodenal switch (Kurian, Thompson, and Davidson 2005). Over time this problem often resolves on its own. High-fat food can also cause loose stools. Diarrhea is not the same as loose stools. Diarrhea is very watery. If you have very watery stools (clear or almost clear) or have more than four bowel movements a day, call your doctor. Otherwise, try these "willing" methods:

- Be patient; it'll take time for your new digestive system to adjust to food.

- Be consistent with writing in your food log so you can eliminate foods that cause problems.

- Eat as low fat as you can.

GAS

Foul-smelling gas is sometimes a problem. Certain foods can cause gas; for example, beans, certain vegetables, and milk cause gas for some people. Use your food log to determine which foods are causing the gas. It's usually possible to control gas by staying away from problem foods (Kurian, Thompson, and Davidson 2005).

Stomach Problems

Common stomach problems after WLS include nausea or vomiting and difficulty swallowing. While all are uncomfortable, nausea and swallowing problems usually resolve if you're willing to take care of your stomach.

NAUSEA AND VOMITING

Being sick to your stomach is miserable. After WLS, nausea and even vomiting can occur, and they can be caused by:

× Eating too fast

× Not drinking enough water and becoming dehydrated

×   Drinking liquids while eating

×   Eating too much

×   Lying down right after eating

×   Eating high-carbohydrate or high-fat foods (remember, one of the major symptoms of sugar dumping is nausea)

In addition to the stated causes, some people find that red meat causes nausea. Food intolerance is an individual matter, so you may find that certain foods just don't agree with your new stomach. Eat slowly, and stop if you feel sick. Particularly in the beginning, your stomach will be sensitive, so go slowly when eating something new and don't overeat. Remember, depending on the WLS you had, your stomach will be able to hold only 2 to 8 ounces of food (or 57 to 226 grams), and particularly in the beginning, your stomach won't like being overfull.

Severe or constant stomach pain, nausea, or unrelenting vomiting can be a symptom of an ulcer or other serious stomach problem. If you have nausea, pain, or vomiting that doesn't resolve by being careful about what and how you eat, see your doctor.

SWALLOWING

After surgery the opening to your stomach, called a *stoma*, is much smaller than it used to be, meaning that only very small bits of food can pass through. This smaller opening makes swallowing a challenge if you don't chew your food very thoroughly. The need to chew all your food thoroughly can't be stressed enough. Chewing initiates the digestion process and prepares food to pass into your stomach pouch. Hopefully you started practicing thoroughly chewing your food before WLS. Chewing food until all that's left is liquid or mush is a good practice for everything you eat.

Nonchewable pills can be uncomfortable to swallow. Some pills should always be crushed, because the pill won't dissolve in your altered digestive system if left whole. Ask your surgeon which pills should be crushed and try these solutions for swallowing pills:

◆   Try, first. Sometimes it's the fear of swallowing the pills that gets in the way, not your stoma. If the pill gets stuck, drink water to dissolve the pill enough to go down. You may be uncomfortable, but the pill should go down in time.

◆   Ask your prescriber if you can take the medication in liquid form. Some medications are available as a liquid preparation.

◆   Find out from your pharmacist if the pill can be cut or crushed. Some pills have a coating and shouldn't be crushed, so check first.

◆   For pills that can be cut, get a pill cutter, cut the pill in half, and swallow each half separately.

◆   Try taking the pill with a little bit of soft food like fat-free yogurt.

Protecting Your Stomach

Some medications are hard on a surgically altered stomach. Don't use over-the-counter pain relievers like aspirin after surgery. Aspirin is in a drug class called *nonsteroid anti-inflammatory drugs*, often called *NSAIDs*. In general avoid all NSAIDs after WLS. These drugs are hard on the digestive system and can cause bleeding and ulcers (Kurian, Thompson, and Davidson 2005). Most people can take Tylenol (generic: acetaminophen) instead of an NSAID, but check with your doctor for individual advice on what to take.

Over-the-Counter Drugs to Avoid After WLS	
NSAIDs:	In addition to the NSAIDs, avoid:
✗ Advil (generic: ibuprofen)	✗ Alka-Seltzer (generic: ASA, citric acid, and sodium bicarbonate) (remember, no carbonation)
✗ Aleve (generic: naproxen)	
✗ Aspirin	✗ Coricidin (generic: acetaminophen and chlorpheniramine)
✗ Bufferin (generic: aspirin)	
✗ Excedrin (generic: acetaminophen, aspirin, and caffeine)	✗ Cortisone
	✗ Vanquish (generic: acetaminophen, aspirin, caffeine)
✗ Fiorinol (generic: aspirin, butalbital, and caffeine)	
✗ Ibuprofen	
✗ Motrin (generic: ibuprofen)	

WHAT'S NEXT?

You're now eating from a narrower range of foods than you were before surgery, but this doesn't mean you can't enjoy your food. In the next chapter we'll look at enjoying food after WLS through mindful eating.

Chapter 14

Life Without Bread: Mindful Eating for the Rest of Your Life

In this chapter we'll explore eating mindfully for the rest of your life. Mindful eating after WLS means enjoying food while continuing to lose weight or to sustain weight loss if you're at your weight goal. It can be challenging to eat mindfully in social situations where others are enjoying foods that you know aren't compatible with your altered digestive system, so we'll also examine how to cope with food events like barbecues and potlucks.

MINDFUL POSTSURGERY EATING

Eating mindfully means planning and following basic postsurgery nutritional guidelines. Impulsive eating, or eating whatever you want, whenever you feel like it, only leads to problems. Using your self-monitoring food logs to do meal planning is a good way to start enjoying food after surgery. *Meal planning* simply means planning ahead of time what you will eat. Meal planning can help you get enough protein and eat foods you enjoy. You can plan a day or a week ahead, depending on your preference. You probably remember the food pyramid you learned about in school. A food pyramid is a good tool for planning tasty meals. Let's look at foods you can enjoy by examining the post-WLS food pyramid.

What to Eat: Food Pyramid for the Rest of Your Life

The standard food pyramid kids learn about in school provides guidelines for healthy eating when you have a normal digestive system. While the standard food pyramid no longer applies to your altered digestive system, a post-WLS food pyramid has been developed that can guide your food choices (Moizé et al. 2010). In a food pyramid, the base food group is the type of food that should make up most of your calories. While the base of the standard food pyramid is complex carbohydrates, like grains and cereals, you won't be surprised to see that the base of the post–WLS pyramid is protein. We'll start our examination of the post-WLS pyramid with the first level of the pyramid: the protein base. Notice that for each food, there's a guideline for serving size and the number of protein grams in one serving to help you plan for sufficient protein.

Level 1: Base of the Pyramid—Protein

Food Group: Protein, four to six servings a day

Eat 60 to 90 grams of protein every day.

Type	Serving size (grams)	Grams of protein per serving	Tips
Chicken	60	15–19	Don't overcook.
Beef	60	15–20	Avoid fatty or tough meat. Don't overcook.
Pork	60	13–19	Avoid fatty or tough meat. Don't overcook.
Fish ◆ Oily fish ◆ Whitefish	 60 85	 13–18 16–23	Eat oily fish at least three days a week.
Dairy ◆ Hard cheese ◆ Soft cheese ◆ Cottage cheese ◆ Milk ◆ Yogurt ◆ Greek yogurt	 50 80 110 140 115 115	 11–13.5 8–12 19 4–5 4–7 10	Choose low-fat or fat-free cheese and fat-free milk, yogurt, and cottage cheese.
Legumes	80	6–8	Mix beans with cereals and grains.

Eggs			
◆ Large whole	50	6	Mix into soups to add protein.
◆ Egg white	33	4	Mix with a whole egg to boost the protein.

After protein you can eat a small amount of other foods. You may be able to eat only a few bits of these foods, depending on the WLS you had. If you're still losing weight, the serving sizes of these foods (below) is too high, so eat a quarter of a serving or less.

The foods on the rest of the pyramid help make food tasty and colorful, as well as give you a variety of nutrients. The next level of the pyramid is high-fiber, low-calorie foods like vegetables and low-sugar fruits.

Level 2: High-Fiber, Low-Calorie Foods

Food Group: Vegetables, two to three servings a day

Type	Serving size (grams)	Grams of protein per serving	Tips
All kinds	85	1–3	Good source of fiber. Chew well.

Food Group: Fruits, two to three servings a day

Low-sugar fresh fruits	70	1	Check the sugar content. Enjoy small amounts of low-sugar fruits like melons, strawberry, and apples. Avoid high-sugar fruits like grapes, oranges, and apricots.

Level 3 of the post-WLS pyramid is grains and cereals. You'll notice that rice and toast are on the list. You can eat small amounts of rice if it's cooked to the point where the grains are starting to fall apart. Once the grains fall apart, the rice can't absorb more liquid, so it won't expand in your stomach. Bread that's toasted to the point where it can't absorb water is also okay. Avoid soft or lightly toasted bread that can expand in your stomach.

Level 3: Grains and Cereals

Food Group: Grains, cereals, and bread, two servings a day

Type	Serving size (grams)	Grams of protein per serving	Tips
Rice, pasta	90	2–5	Choose whole grains. Rice must be overcooked, until the grains are falling apart. Mix with beans.
Breakfast cereals	30	2–4	Avoid sugared cereals.
Toast	30	2–4	Well toasted: avoid soft bread.

The last level of the pyramid is high-calorie foods, including fats and sweets. Sweets are not good for you, so you won't see them on this list. You do need a very small amount of fat in your diet. Fats that are solid are always a bad idea, which means butter and lard are out. Stay with liquid fats, like olive oil.

Level 4: Fats

Food Group: Oil, two servings a day

Type	Serving size (grams)	Grams of protein per serving	Tips
Olive oil	6 (1 teaspoon)	0	Choose vegetable oils. Olive oil is a very good choice. Avoid saturated fats, like butter.
Sunflower oil	6 (1 teaspoon)	0	Good alternative to olive oil.

Adhering to the pyramid guidelines will allow you to stay healthy and keep the weight off. Remember to also consult your nutritional tool, particularly when trying new foods. If you're having difficulty with portion sizes, use a food scale to help you keep your grams per serving low.

Putting a Meal Together

Because mindful eating is about health and enjoyment, let's look at how to put together meals that are tasty while following the pyramid. Next, review what Josie eats for breakfast and lunch in the left-hand column of the following table. Do you think she eats enough protein at these two meals? How does she use high-fiber, low-protein foods to make the meals interesting? Josie needs at least 60 grams of protein a day. In the upper-right-hand box, plan a dinner for her that gives her the remaining protein she needs while following the pyramid recommendations for other foods.

Breakfast: One whole egg and one egg white, scrambled with chopped spinach, low-fat cheese, and finely chopped green onion Protein: ✓ Eggs: 10 g ✓ Cheese: 12 g *Total protein: 22 g*	**Dinner:** Plan Josie's dinner: _____ _____ _____ _____
Lunch: Half a piece of toast with yogurt, chicken, and strawberries (finely chopped chicken mixed with chopped strawberries, celery powder, and fat-free yogurt) Protein: ✓ Chicken: 15 g ✓ Yogurt: 4 g *Total protein: 19 g*	Fill in Josie's totals for the day: Pyramid base—protein: _____ grams Level 2—high-fiber, low-protein: _____ servings Level 3—grains and cereals: _____ servings Level 4—fats: _____ servings

Was it easy to complete Josie's day? Hopefully you gave her at least 19 to 20 grams of protein for dinner. Did you add low-sugar fruit and a vegetable to make her dinner colorful and tasty? Just eating protein can be boring, so one of the roles low-protein food plays is enhancing the taste and look of foods. Now that we have examined what to eat, let's look at how to eat mindfully.

How to Eat Mindfully

Eating mindfully is as much about how you eat as what you eat. Here are six basic rules for how to eat mindfully after WLS:

◆ Eat slowly. You've probably been practicing eating slowly for a while now. After WLS, eating quickly can lead to pain and difficulty swallowing. In addition to experiencing pain, now that you are eating much less volume, eating quickly will leave you feeling as if you missed the experience of eating.

◆ Don't talk and eat at the same time. You probably heard this rule from your mother or grandmother, and it's a good one. Talking and eating at the same time is more than impolite. If you're talking, you might not chew enough and might try to swallow food that's too big to pass through your stoma. And you'll miss out on the experience of tasting your food. This doesn't mean you shouldn't socialize over food; just do one thing at a time. If you're chewing, chew. If you're talking, talk. Don't multitask while eating.

◆ Always sit at a table to eat. Don't eat on the go or standing up. Make the meal an event.

◆ While you chew, focus on noticing taste and texture. Consider the flavors as you move the food around in your mouth. Notice how the texture of the food changes as you chew. And don't forget about smell. Smell is important to taste, so using herbs that smell good and taste good can really enhance your food.

◆ Make your food look good. Use nice tableware and garnishes, and add some color to your food. Just a little finely chopped parsley or green onion can really make a difference.

◆ Use self-monitoring when you encounter problems. Self-monitoring is the best way to troubleshoot eating problems.

FOOD EVENTS

From Thanksgiving dinner, potlucks, and barbecues to intimate dinners for two, eating is often a social activity. Problems with eating at food events include:

◆ Eating or drinking foods that are high in fat or carbohydrates

◆ Grazing or nibbling on food throughout the event

◆ Overeating or bingeing

◆ Skipping a meal or avoiding eating altogether

◆ Missing the event rather than facing the menu

Recall the last social event you attended that included food, and answer these questions:

How much food was at the event? _____

_____

How important was food to the event? _____

_____

Were you expected to eat, or did you feel pressured to eat? If yes, explain: _____

_____

_____

How did it feel to be faced with food you couldn't eat? _____

_____

Did you eat or drink something you knew was bad for you? If yes, what did you eat or drink?

_____

_____

Do you have a food event coming up that you're concerned about? If yes, what are you concerned about? (At the end of this chapter, you'll have the opportunity to plan an effective strategy for this event.)

_____

_____

When Josie answers these questions, she realizes she is in the habit of nibbling on food she knows is unhealthy when she goes to a food event. At first it doesn't seem to be a problem, because she doesn't experience sugar dumping and only "tastes the food," but over time, with each food event she attends, she eats a little more. Mark develops a different problem. He doesn't eat food that's unhealthy; instead he avoids eating altogether, which results in skipping meals and not getting enough protein for the day. Both of these social eating issues are common postsurgery problems. Enjoying social events involving food after WLS means being willing to plan ahead and change your social behavior.

Let's look at how to handle different types of food events. Broadly speaking, we can divide food events into these categories:

- Family dinners, like Thanksgiving dinner or dinner at a relative's home

- Celebratory events, like weddings

- Barbecues and potlucks

- Work events

- Intimate dinners for two

Let's look at tips for dealing with each type of event, starting with family events.

Family Events

Family events can be easy or difficult depending on your family and your relationship with family members. Assuming you have an understanding family and good relationships, an effective way to deal with family events is to talk about what you can eat prior to the event. It's also helpful to offer to bring a dish you know you can eat. It's best to avoid surprises, so if you suspect your favorite aunt will bring your favorite dessert, let her know before the event.

Celebratory Events

Events such as weddings, anniversary parties, and birthdays can be good occasions to eat mindfully if the food is served buffet style, because there are usually lots of choices.

If you follow a few rules, buffets are good venues for eating well:

- ◆ Check out the buffet first to plan what you will eat.

- ◆ Use a dessert plate, not a dinner plate.

- ◆ Put lean protein on your plate first and then add vegetables.

- ◆ Avoid anything fried or anything in a sauce.

- ◆ Avoid salads, which are often drenched in dressing.

- ◆ Go to the buffet once; no seconds.

- ◆ Sit far away from the dessert table.

If it's a sit-down meal, try to view the menu in advance. Normally some kind of meat or fish will be served. If the event's at a hotel or restaurant, ask the server to bring you the meat without sauce and a vegetable side dish without butter. Remember, food allergies are common, so you probably won't be the only one making a special request.

ALTERNATIVE WAYS TO CELEBRATE

Sometimes, finding an alternative way to celebrate that doesn't focus on food is a good option. Megan and her family decide to volunteer on Thanksgiving rather than cook a large meal for the family. This helps Megan prepare for WLS and helps her mother, who is post-WLS and concerned about weight regain. Josie decides to celebrate her birthday by walking a 5K race. She spends three months increasing her endurance in anticipation of her birthday walk. Though she finishes toward the end of the group of walkers, for Josie it's an important accomplishment. Afterward she says, "It was the best birthday present I could have given myself." Next, write your ideas for celebrating without food and include an idea for the next event you plan to celebrate.

My ideas for celebrating without food:

Use money I would normally have spent on a big dinner out to buy a special outfit instead.

The next event is: _____.

I plan to celebrate without food by: _____

Barbecues and Potlucks

Barbecues and potlucks can be fun food events as long as you stay away from the high-fat potato salad or sugar-loaded desserts. There's almost always some kind of meat or fish at barbecues and potlucks, so protein isn't usually a problem. Avoid barbecue sauces, which often contain a lot of sugar. Always bring a protein dish you can eat, making sure it's something you really like, in case it's the only dish you can eat, and try the previous buffet tips.

Work Events

If the food is served buffet style, follow the previous buffet tips. Try to get involved in the planning and ask about healthier choices. If your company has an employee wellness committee, get the committee to advocate for a healthy menu. You may find that your coworkers also appreciate a work event that incorporates healthy food choices.

Intimate Dinners for Two

Depending on the relationship, dinners for two can be easy or complicated. Weight loss gives Josie the confidence she needs to try online dating. The first dinner date Josie has is a food disaster. She doesn't pick the restaurant and finds herself meeting her date at a restaurant that specializes, in Josie's words, in "fried everything." Feeling too embarrassed to tell him she is post-WLS, Josie tries to eat from the menu but learns a hard lesson when she experiences loose stools a few hours later. The next time she plans a dinner date, she explains that she is on a special diet and asks if it's okay if she picks the restaurant. Needless to say, the next dating experience is more positive, and Josie can concentrate on getting to know her date rather than the menu. Try these tips for intimate dinners:

- Talk about food beforehand.

- Pick the restaurant or do the cooking.

◆ If you're having dinner with someone you don't know well, consider what to disclose. If you aren't comfortable disclosing that you're post-WLS, just say you follow a special diet. Lots of people follow special diets for lots of reasons; you don't have to disclose the reason for your special diet.

◆ If your dinner partner is someone close to you who doesn't understand the importance of your being careful about what you eat, educate her.

Your Next Event

Review the previous question about your next social event. In the following box, use what you've learned in this chapter to plan how to deal with this event.

I can do the following to help me enjoy both the food and the people:

WHAT'S NEXT?

Poor body image is common in people who are obese. And because many thin people also suffer from poor body image, losing weight won't automatically improve your body image (Cash 1997). In the next chapter we'll look at body image and how to feel good about your body.

Chapter 15

Improving Your Body Image with ACCEPT

Body image is how you think and feel about your body. Given the fact that obesity has a negative effect on body image, you probably didn't have a good body image before losing weight (Sarwer et al. 2008a). Loose skin, a less than 100 percent excess-weight loss, and years of disliking your body may contribute to your negative view of your body. The good news is you can improve your body image. Improving how you think and feel about your body doesn't mean loving everything about it. Improving your body image means learning to accept what you don't like and feel satisfied with the body you have right now. Even if you're still losing weight or planning surgery to remove excess skin, you can benefit from improving your body image. Body-image improvement is an ongoing task, and this is the same reality that naturally thin people face. Our bodies change as we age, so body-image work is a lifetime task. Let's look at how you can improve your body image with the acronym ACCEPT, in which each letter stands for action you can take to improve your body image.

ACCEPT

A—Accept

C—Care

C—Compliment

E—End judgment

P—Pursue

T—Take Risks

ACCEPT

If it has been more than a few months since your surgery, you've probably already lost enough weight to change the size and shape of your body. Change requires acceptance, even if it's the change you've been hoping for. If you've been obese most of your life, living in a thinner body is a dramatic change. If you were thin before you became obese, your body probably isn't back to the pre-obese one you enjoyed when you were younger. Regardless of whether you used to be thin or you have been obese since childhood, the reality is that there's probably something about your body that you're struggling with. Check any of these common realities you've struggled with:

- ☐ Disappointment in weight loss

- ☐ Sagging or loose skin

- ☐ Disappointment in body shape

- ☐ Looking older

- ☐ Hair loss

The good news is that even if you checked off all five realities, you can improve your body image. Let's start with the first step in ACCEPT: accept.

*A*CCEPT: Accept

To accept means to be willing to learn to accept your body with flaws. One of the realities that can be hard to accept is your amount of weight loss. In chapter 1 we discussed realistic expectations for weight loss. In chapter 12 you developed your weight loss goal. If you didn't make it to your goal weight or you're holding out hope for 100 percent excess-weight loss, you might be disappointed. Part of accepting that your weight loss may not have made you into a thin person is defining your success beyond the number on the scale. What *quality-of-life successes* has losing weight brought you? In the following box, define your success.

Defining My Success Beyond Weight Loss

Think back to all the reasons you had WLS. Did you really have WLS just to wear a smaller size? Why did you have the surgery? _____

_____

What physical activities can you do now that you couldn't do before? _____

_____

_____

What health problems were interfering with your life that are now resolved or improved?

_____

_____

Next, check all your successes:

☐ Improved sleep   ☐ More confidence in social situations

☐ Less joint or back pain   ☐ Improved relationships

☐ Ability to fit into seats   ☐ More energy

☐ Improved walking   ☐ Enjoying moving your body

☐ Feeling better about yourself ☐ Increased occupational opportunities

☐ Other: _____   ☐ Other: _____

LOOSE SKIN

About two thirds of people who have WLS report significant loose skin in one or more areas (Sarwer et al. 2008a). Loose and sagging skin on arms, bellies, breasts, buttocks, and necks is common. Loose skin affects body shape, making it necessary to buy larger-size clothing to accommodate the excess skin. Many people also feel that loose skin makes them look older. A round, plump face is a young look, whereas a thinner face with loose skin at the neck, or jowls, can be aging. In addition to the cosmetic aspects of loose skin, excess skin can cause physical or medical problems. For example, excess skin around your middle can make it difficult to bend over, and you can have skin problems under skin folds. You have two choices for dealing with loose skin: have excess skin removed surgically, or learn to live with your loose skin. Both choices require acceptance.

Plastic Surgery: Plastic surgery has a positive effect on body image and improves quality of life for most people who choose to have skin removed after WLS (Van der Beek et al. 2010). Reasons to have skin removed include:

◆ Improved appearance

- ◆ Improved physical functioning, like bending over

- ◆ Improved personal hygiene

- ◆ Resolved skin problems, like rashes under skin folds

Check with your insurance company to see if skin removal is covered under your benefits. *Abdominoplasty*, or removal of abdominal skin, is the surgery most often covered by insurance. Hanging abdominal skin that's bad enough to interfere with walking or that causes other medical problems, like infections and rashes under the skin flap, may meet your insurance company's definition of medical necessity. Hanging skin in other areas of the body, like arms and legs, is usually not covered, because there are rarely medical reasons for the removal.

While plastic surgery to remove excess skin can have a positive effect on the way you feel about your body, it still requires acceptance. Removal of hanging skin on some areas of the body, like arms, requires long incisions, which can mean unsightly scars.

Before you decide to have plastic surgery for loose skin, you'll need to accept these facts (check any facts you feel are difficult to accept):

- ☐ You may have to pay out of pocket for the plastic surgery.

- ☐ Skin removal surgery typically causes more pain than WLS.

- ☐ Depending on the amount of skin being removed and location of the excess skin, surgery for skin removal can take much longer than WLS.

- ☐ Scarring is a common problem. Scars running the length of your arms may not look that much better to you than flapping arm skin.

- ☐ Healing takes time, and you'll have swelling for a while afterward. It can take months for swelling to diminish, depending on the surgery you had.

- ☐ Even if you want to have several surgeries at once, that may not be possible, and you might need multiple separate surgeries to have all your excess skin removed. This means more time off work.

Finally, carefully choose your plastic surgeon. Removing loose skin after WLS is not the same as having a little nip and tuck. Work with a plastic surgeon who's familiar with the problems of removing large amounts of skin.

Living with Loose Skin: If you choose not to have skin removed or not to have *all* your loose skin removed, there are undergarments that can help you live with loose skin. In fact the number of choices in foundation undergarments for women and men has increased in recent years, and it's worth trying a few. But in the end, most people face the issue of acceptance. In the following table, write where you have loose skin, and rank your willingness to accept the excess skin or the effects of plastic surgery for each area, using a scale from 0 to 5, where 0 means you're unwilling to work on acceptance and 5 means you're very willing to work on acceptance.

Loose Skin Acceptance Ranking		
Area of loose skin	*Acceptance ranking for living with loose skin*	*Acceptance ranking for plastic surgery effects*

Examine your rankings for each area. If you ranked an area 1 or 2 for loose skin on the acceptance scale and ranked plastic surgery acceptance at 3, 4, or 5, consider plastic surgery for that area. If, on the other hand, your plastic surgery rankings are 1 or 2 for acceptance, learning to accept your loose skin may be the way to go. As you work on acceptance of loose skin or acceptance of plastic surgery, keep in mind that acceptance isn't something that happens all at once, nor does acceptance mean you'll learn to like your loose skin. Acceptance means coming to conclusions like:

◆ Although I'll never like having loose skin, the benefits of weight loss are worth it.

◆ There are parts of my body I like.

◆ The reasons not to have skin removed are more important to me than dealing with the loose skin.

◆ I can accept that having plastic surgery means accepting scarring.

ACCEPT: Care for Your Body

Caring for your body helps you feel better about how your body looks. You're already caring for your body by losing weight. When you care for your body, you're sending the message that your body is worth caring for. You can care for your body by doing relaxation exercises, getting a pedicure, or doing other body-caring activities. From the following list, check any body-caring activities you plan to do, adding at least two activities of your own. Commit to doing at least three of your body-caring activities every week.

- [ ] Do relaxation exercises.
- [ ] Get a pedicure or manicure.
- [ ] Get your hair done.
- [ ] Sit in the sun and enjoy its warmth on your skin.
- [ ] Put on clothes that fit your new body and notice how the smaller size feels.
- [ ] See a fashion consultant to learn how to dress your new body.
- [ ] Soak in a hot tub or Jacuzzi.
- [ ] Start wearing makeup.
- [ ] Take up dancing.
- [ ] Take a hot shower or bubble bath.
- [ ] Other: _____
- [ ] Other: _____

CLOTHING

How we dress expresses how we feel about our bodies, and one way to take care of your body is to wear clothes that fit you, are fashionable, and express your personality. Wardrobe neglect is common in people living with obesity. Josie, whose outgoing personality is consistent with a fashionable, "edgy" style, first arrived at my office in a well-worn flowered shirt and black pants. Josie's experience of being unable to find fashionable clothes left her feeling defeated about her wardrobe. Since her WLS, Josie does very little shopping, explaining, "I'm waiting until I get to my goal weight to get new clothes." While Josie's attitude about her clothes might not seem important, it interferes with her adjustment to her new body. The large clothes she wears hide her weight loss, making her feel bigger than she is. Wearing clothes that fit is a way to care for your body, adjust to its changing size, and express yourself. If you're waiting until you lose additional weight to shop, or if you're "saving the fat clothes, just in case," it's time to get rid of the clothes that don't fit and go shopping.

Post-WLS Clothing Exchange

It can be expensive to buy several wardrobes as your size shrinks. Some WLS support groups host clothing exchanges. This can be a good way to get rid of clothes that are in good shape but are too big and to receive clothes that fit.

ACCEPT: Compliment

Many of us get compliments about our appearance, only to dismiss them. One way to feel better about your body is to let others help you by accepting their compliments. When you get a compliment about your body, write it down. A body compliment can be anything from "Your hair looks good" to "You look healthier." Write down the compliments you receive that are helpful. Ignore comments that reinforce unhealthy behavior, like "You've lost so much weight; you can have dessert this one time."

Write the compliments in a notebook or journal. The key here is to write down the compliment just as it was intended, without adding to or taking away from what was said. For example, if someone says, "You look good," write it down, without taking away from the compliment by adding, "How can she say that? I'm still fat." In other words, accept the compliment as it's given. In the next box, write at least two compliments you've received.

Compliments I've received since my surgery:

ACCEPT: End Judgment

Negative body judgment is a common habit. If you're disappointed in or dislike a part of your body, it's easy to engage in critical body judgment, like "My face looks so wrinkled and old" or "My shape is lumpy and ugly." It's common for negative body judgments to include assumptions about how the rest of the world responds to our bodies. For example, "My shape is lumpy and ugly" might be paired with "and people think I look bad." What have you been judgmental about? Next, write down your negative body judgments.

My negative body judgments:

Before you work on changing your judgments, let's look at Mark's negative body judgments:

◆ *I'm still fat; no women will want me with the fat and loose skin.*

◆ *My face looks so old, I'll never get a date.*

What did you notice about Mark's judgments? It's common for judgmental thinking to have a theme. In Mark's case, the theme is that his loose skin makes him look old and fat, which Mark thinks means not being attractive to the opposite sex. Loose skin can add girth, so even though Mark has had good weight loss, his loose skin makes him look a little bigger than he is, and his face has more winkles. Now let's look at how Mark ends his judgmental thinking by focusing on being realistic and factual:

- ◆ *My body is smaller. I lost a lot of weight, but the loose skin has added wrinkles and some bulk. A woman who's interested in me will have to accept that the loose skin is a good trade-off for being with a man who's healthy and active.*

- ◆ *I might look a little older, but I'm healthier and more confident; some women may like that.*

Notice that Mark doesn't change his thinking with unrealistic statements like *I look young and fit, as I did when I was playing football* or *Lots of women want to date me.* These statements aren't factual or realistic. It's a fact that Mark looks older and has some loose skin. And it's a fact that Mark may have to put some effort into finding a woman who's a good match. But it's also a fact that Mark is now a healthy, active person, and it's realistic that he can find a woman who will want to spend time with him. Now it's time for you to change the negative judgmental thoughts you wrote in the previous box. Remember to be realistic and stick to the facts. Leave out the judgment.

My "end judgment" thoughts:

ACCE**P**T: Pursue a Healthy Body

Pursuing a healthy body and good body image means eating, exercising, and getting enough sleep. Follow these simple rules:

Eat regularly: Eat three meals a day, making sure to get enough protein and take your vitamins.

Exercise: Exercise is a must. Movement helps your brain experience your new body.

Get enough sleep: Eight to ten hours of sleep each night is ideal for most people. Many people overeat when feeling tired, so work on improving your sleep. If you have problems with getting enough sleep, check out the resources section in the back of this book for suggestions on improving sleep.

ACCEP**T**: Take Risks

Taking risks builds confidence. Taking a risk by trying new physical activities can help you have confidence in your body. You don't have to jump out of an airplane or take up deep-sea diving to take a physical risk. Taking dance lessons or completing a 5K walk or run is a risk if you didn't or couldn't do these things before. Megan takes a risk by joining a softball team after her WLS. Finding out that she can run, along with the relationships she develops with the other team members, gives Megan confidence in her body and herself. Review the following physical activities (check any you plan to try, and add two ideas of your own):

- ☐ Walking longer distances
- ☐ Running
- ☐ Bicycling
- ☐ Surfing
- ☐ Dancing
- ☐ Hiking
- ☐ Yoga
- ☐ Completing a walk or run (5K, 10K, half marathon, or marathon)
- ☐ Taking up a sport you never tried or haven't done in a while: _____
- ☐ Other: _____
- ☐ Other: _____

PUTTING IT ALL TOGETHER

We accept change, not because we like the change but because rejecting change doesn't work. Now it's time to put what you've learned from ACCEPT into an activity that focuses on the body issue you've struggled with the most. Review the list of common realities at the beginning of this chapter and, for this activity, use the issue that has been the hardest for you to accept.

Acceptance Activity, Part 1

The body issue I struggle with the most is: _____.

1. List all the things you don't like. Make sure to end judgment by making the list factual. For example, write, "The skin on my arms hangs down when I raise them," not "The loose skin on my arms makes me look ugly."

    ☑ I don't like:

2. Now list your offsets. An offset is a benefit of your weight loss. For example, an offset might be "My diabetes is completely resolved." Now list the offsets:

    ☑ I don't like _____, but I like these offsets:

3. List all the things you like about your body now that you didn't like before. Focus on physical appearance. As with the first list, state the facts; for example, say, "My legs are thinner."

    ☑ I like these changes in my body:

Now you're ready to write an acceptance statement. An acceptance statement acknowledges what you like and don't like about your body, paired with a commitment to learning to accept the body you have right now. Let's look at examples of acceptance statements.

Josie's Acceptance Statement: "I don't like that I haven't lost all the weight I want to lose, but I am much healthier and no longer have prediabetes. I can learn to accept this body and enjoy my good health while I work on losing a little more weight."

Mark's Acceptance Statement: "I don't like the loose skin, but it's worth the loose skin to be able to walk again. I know I can't go back thirty years and have the body from my football days, but I really enjoy being able to move around and walk without a cane. I can learn to accept this healthier, more mobile body, loose skin and all."

Megan's Acceptance Statement: "I might never be as thin as some girls, but I've lost more weight than I ever did before. Now I can shop for clothes in some regular stores. I can learn to accept this body."

As you may have noticed, an acceptance statement isn't unrealistic, nor is it a positive affirmation like "I'm thin and beautiful." It's a statement that acknowledges the good with the bad and includes a commitment to work on acceptance. An easy way to start is with what you don't like, followed by what has improved, and, last, your commitment to learn body acceptance. Now it's time to write your acceptance statement.

Acceptance Activity, Part 2: My Acceptance Statement

I don't like _____ .

But now, _____ .

I can learn to accept _____ .

WHAT'S NEXT?

Inadequate weight loss and weight regain have become two of the disappointments of WLS. Before the increase in surgically assisted weight loss, it was assumed that everyone would lose an adequate amount of weight and weight regain would be rare. Unfortunately inadequate weight loss and regain after WLS isn't rare, with higher risk of inadequate weight loss and regain with gastric banding. In the next chapter we'll look at how to achieve adequate weight loss and how to prevent or reverse weight regain.

Chapter 16

Solutions for Inadequate Weight Loss and Weight Regain

Inadequate weight loss and weight regain are postsurgery problems that should be addressed quickly. If you stopped losing weight before reaching 50 percent of your excess weight (40 percent if you had gastric banding), you're experiencing inadequate weight loss. If you've regained more than a few pounds before your weight stabilized, you're experiencing weight regain that, if unstopped, can lead to regain of every pound you lost with WLS. It's not uncommon for these two problems to occur together, but luckily the solutions are the same for both problems.

After achieving a 40 to 70 percent excess-weight loss, it's normal to regain a little weight after the first year or two before your weight stabilizes (Shah, Simha, and Garg 2006). An example of a common pattern would be an initial loss of 70 percent of excess weight after RNYGB, and then gaining a little weight in the second or third year before stabilizing at a 60 or 65 percent overall loss. Unfortunately, for some people, weight regain continues. Even worse, if you experience inadequate weight loss and start to regain weight, it won't be long before you end up at the weight you started with. This is the situation Josie finds herself in when she starts to regain after losing only 35 percent of her weight with RNYGB. Josie is able to get back on track, and so can you, if you find yourself in this situation. The good news is that most of the reasons and all of the solutions for inadequate weight loss and regain are under your control. The key is to take action quickly and not wait until you've regained most of your lost weight. Let's start by examining the causes of inadequate weight loss and weight regain.

THE CAUSES OF INADEQUATE WEIGHT LOSS AND WEIGHT REGAIN

There are five common causes of inadequate weight loss and regain after WLS, but only two of the five causes are beyond your control. The causes are:

- A drop in BMR

- Increased efficiency in calorie absorption

- Increased calorie intake

- Problem eating

- Insufficient exercise

We'll start with the two causes you can't control, but remember, even if you don't have control over the cause, you control the solution.

Decrease in BMR and Increase in Efficiency

A number of studies have looked at basal metabolic rate (BMR) after surgery. While we know that BMR increases after surgery, sometimes that increase isn't maintained. Why BMR changes aren't sustained isn't completely understood, but it's clear that WLS won't automatically lead to a long-term BMR increase for everyone who has surgery (Shah, Simha, and Garg 2006).

A related problem is a change in absorption. If you had a WLS that impairs absorption, it's possible for your body to become more efficient at absorbing calories over time (Kurian, Thompson, and Davidson 2005). As with BMR changes, it's not known exactly why increased absorption occurs.

Because the decrease in BMR and increased absorption rarely occur in the first twelve to twenty-four months after surgery, it's important to work on achieving all or most of your expected weight loss during those early months. It's still possible to lose weight after twenty-four months, but you may need to work harder to lose.

It can be tempting to blame your inadequate loss or regain on these poorly understood physical causes, but with the exception of minor regain, BMR and absorption changes probably don't cause most inadequate weight loss or gain. So before you jump to conclusions, carefully review your self-monitoring food log and ask yourself these questions:

- Have you increased your total calories over time?

- Are you eating the wrong foods?

- Have you decreased your physical activity or stopped exercising?

If you answered no to all three questions, it's possible your BMR has dropped or your body has become more efficient at absorbing the calories. If you answered yes or "sometimes" to any of these questions, there's probably a cause to your inadequate weight loss or weight regain that's not related to BMR or absorption.

SOLUTION

If you've lost adequate weight and your weight regain is minor (say five to ten pounds) and doesn't continue, you may want to accept the situation. Adjust your five-pound target weight range accordingly. However, if you didn't lose enough weight or your regain continues, you need to take action. The solution is to decrease calorie intake and increase your physical activity. Be very careful about carbohydrates and liquid calories; these are easily absorbed. Increase exercise to increase your BMR.

INCREASING CALORIC INTAKE

Increasing calories will lead to inadequate weight loss and weight regain and is probably the most common cause of these problems. Respond to these questions:

- ◆ Have you stopped planning meals and started eating whatever's handy?
- ◆ Are you eating foods that are high in carbohydrates, sugar, or fat?
- ◆ Have you been overeating or eating foods that can stretch your stoma or stomach?
- ◆ Are you drinking a lot of calories?
- ◆ Have you stopped self-monitoring?

If you answered yes to any of these questions, you've probably increased your calories. Many people increase fat and carbohydrate grams over time—without even being aware of it. It turns out that when we compare people who regain weight to those who don't, we see a difference in the percentage of calories coming from fat, carbohydrate, and sugar (Moizé et al. 2010). As the consumption of lean protein goes down and that of fat, carbohydrates, and sugar goes up, the total calories eaten also tends to go up, and you gain weight. Another way to increase your calories is to drink them. It's easy to drink calorie-rich drinks like milkshakes or juice that don't stay in the stomach long. These drinks provide calories that are easily absorbed. If you had gastric banding, drinking calories can quickly lead to little or no weight loss or complete weight regain.

In addition to drinking calories, a factor that makes it easier to consume additional calories is stretching your stomach pouch or stoma. Stretching occurs with overeating or eating foods that expand in the stomach. The simple fact is the larger your stoma or stomach, the more you can eat.

SOLUTION

You may have started to think you can eat normally, which is a willful kind of thinking. Carefully review chapter 8 to increase your cognitive restraint of eating, plus chapters 12 and 13. It's time to start taking care of your altered digestive system. Make self-monitoring a habit. If you have stretched your stoma or stomach, you can consult your surgeon—sometimes there's a surgical solution—but remember, what you stretch once, you can stretch twice, so change the way you eat *first*.

Problem Eating

It's possible to slip back into problem eating behaviors. Bingeing or grazing on food all day after WLS is an all-too-common problem. Respond to these questions:

◆ Are you skipping meals?

◆ Are you snacking or grazing all day?

◆ Have you started to binge-eat?

◆ Are you struggling with emotional triggers?

If you answered yes to any of these questions, you could be engaging in problem eating or even disordered eating. In the first two years, it may be physically difficult to eat large amounts of food, but you can still eat in a way that's a binge in everything but size, and over time you'll find you can eat larger and larger amounts. Post-WLS binge behavior is defined as follows

◆ Eating until you're uncomfortably full

◆ Eating food that contains little protein

◆ Feeling guilty or upset afterward

In addition to bingeing, grazing on small amounts of food all day leads to inadequate weight loss or weight regain.

SOLUTION

Practice self-monitoring and review chapters 6 through 9. If you can't get your eating under control, seek professional help. Continuing to engage in problem eating behaviors can lead to losing little weight or regaining every pound you lost. A common trigger for problem eating behaviors after WLS is our old friend, the emotional trigger. Use self-monitoring to see if you're using food to deal with emotions. See an eating-disorder specialist if you can't get your eating under control on your own. Don't wait too long to seek help. Remember, it's usually harder to lose weight the second time around.

Lack of Exercise

If you stop exercising, you'll interfere with weight loss, or you'll regain weight. Staying active is very important. Answer these questions about your activity level:

◆ Have you abandoned your exercise plan?

◆   Are you exercising fewer than four times a week?

◆   Do you exercise less now than you did before your surgery?

If you answered yes to any of the questions, you probably aren't exercising enough. Regular exercise is very important in weight loss and weight-loss maintenance (Shah, Simha, and Garg 2006).

SOLUTION

Increase your physical activity. If you don't have an exercise plan, develop one. If you have a plan but haven't been following it, start following your plan. Review chapter 5.

Ten Things a Surgeon Wants You to Remember
by Arnold D. Salzberg, MD

1. Bariatric surgery is not a fad, a quick fix, or a diet supplement. All such surgeries can be circumvented. Keep in mind that this endeavor is a lifelong commitment, the most important part of which is you. The surgery is merely a tool to help you succeed, with the objective of adding valuable years to your life!

2. Take your self-monitoring food log to your dietitian or doctor, so adjustments can be made. Patients who keep food logs are the most successful at getting to their goal weight.

3. Keep your food separated from that of the rest of the people in the house. It cuts down on temptation.

4. The most important willpower moment of the week is when you go to the grocery. Avoid buying food that's not good for you, to help you keep from eating something unhealthy at night, when it's hard to resist temptation.

5. Set a time limit for your meals. Give yourself fifteen to thirty minutes to eat breakfast, lunch, or dinner, and you'll find you're eating until you're no longer hungry, not until you're stuffed.

6. Eat as few calories as you can while still getting enough protein.

7. Keep your carbohydrate total to no more than 20 grams per day.

8. Stay hydrated. Drink at least 64 ounces of water a day.

9. Chew food thoroughly. For most food, this means chewing twenty to thirty times.

10. Take your vitamins. Crush them first if you've been instructed to do so.

LOSING TOO MUCH WEIGHT

Occasionally, excess weight loss results from WLS. While this is not a common problem, if your BMI drops to 18 or lower, see your doctor to make sure your weight loss isn't due to a medical problem. If excess weight loss is due to not eating enough, seek the help of an eating-disorder specialist. Extremely low weight is dangerous. It's essential that you gain enough weight to move your BMI into the normal range.

DEPRESSION AND ANXIETY

Feeling depressed or anxious can interfere with losing weight and keeping it off. If you had a history of depressive or anxiety disorders before WLS and you think you're feeling the way you did when you were diagnosed, get help right away. If you don't have a history of psychological problems but are feeling down or anxious, return to chapter 9 and take the Depressive Disorder/Anxiety Disorder Screen again. If you answer yes to one or more questions for depression or anxiety, or if you feel hopeless and think about dying, see a mental health professional.

WHAT'S NEXT?

You've put a lot of time and energy into weight loss. You'll probably have to watch your weight for the rest of your life. This means being careful about what you eat to ensure that you eat enough protein and care for your altered digestive system. But your life doesn't have to revolve around your weight and WLS. In the next chapter we'll look at how to live your life beyond WLS.

Chapter 17

What Next? Building a New Life

Congratulations! You have put a lot of time and effort into improving your health and reaching your compelling goal. Continue checking your weight regularly so you can take immediate steps if it exceeds your five-pound range. And of course, exercise, eating enough protein, and taking vitamins should be part of your routine for the rest of your life. But now, your focus can move from losing weight and resolving obesity-related health conditions to setting new goals in order to build a new life that goes beyond WLS. Sometimes there are beliefs that hold people back from moving on and building a new life after WLS. Even if you reached your weight loss and compelling goals, there may be beliefs about obesity or weight loss that are holding you back, so we'll start by looking at those beliefs.

BELIEFS THAT HOLD YOU BACK

We learned in chapter 7 that how you think can lead to eating problems. Similarly what you believe about obesity and weight loss can hold you back from living a life beyond WLS. Check your obesity or weight-loss beliefs (add at least two of your own):

- [ ] Naturally thin people have it all.
- [ ] The first thing people notice is how fat someone is.
- [ ] Overweight people are less likeable.
- [ ] I'm a failure if I don't lose 100 percent of my excess weight.
- [ ] If people knew I used to be fat, they would like me less.
- [ ] My weight has influenced everything that's happened in my life.

☐ I've lost weight, so now I have to be successful (perfect).

☐ I'll never be thin enough to fit society's image of attractive, so I'll never be satisfied with my body.

☐ Other: _____

☐ Other: _____

How many beliefs did you check? Now it's time to challenge these beliefs. Before you write your challenges, let's look at how Megan challenges some of her beliefs.

Talking Back—Megan	
Megan's Belief	*Megan's Challenge*
Naturally thin people have it all.	*No one has it all; I know thin people who have problems too.*
The first thing people notice is how fat someone is.	*I'm superfocused on weight, but many people aren't. My friends on the softball team see me as a good hitter, not a fat girl.*
I'm a failure if I don't lose 100 percent of my excess weight.	*I may never lose 100 percent, but what makes me succeed in life is more than what the scale says. I'm active and healthy; I can move on with my life and achieve other things, like earning my college degree.*
My weight has influenced everything that has happened in my life.	*It's true that my weight has affected my life, but other things have affected my life too, like being good at math and having a family that supports me.*

Notice how Megan uses facts and her experiences to challenge her beliefs. Now it's time for you to challenge your beliefs. The challenge should be something you think you can believe, so stay away from challenges like "No one notices how much other people weigh." That's unrealistic, and you probably won't believe such a challenge.

Talking Back	
Belief	*Challenge*
Naturally thin people have it all.	
The first thing people notice is how fat someone is.	
Overweight people are less likeable.	
I'm a failure if I don't lose 100 percent of my weight.	
If people knew I used to be fat, they would like me less.	
My weight has influenced everything that has happened in my life.	
I lost a lot of weight, so now I have to be successful (perfect).	
I'll never be thin enough to fit society's image of attractive, so I will never be satisfied with my body.	
Other: _____	_____
Other: _____	_____

Challenging beliefs takes more than one activity. As you move on with your life, you'll probably have to challenge your obesity and weight-loss beliefs again. Keep working on challenging beliefs that hold you back as you move on with your life.

WHAT'S CHANGED?

There are many ways WLS changes lives. We've spent a lot of time discussing how surgery changes your digestive system and how weight loss can help resolve medical conditions like diabetes. Now it's time to consider how the process of losing weight with WLS has changed your life over and above improving your health. What aspects of your life have changed? Have there been any surprises? Josie is surprised to find that she likes clothes. Before her weight loss, she wore whatever she found that fit, without thinking about fashion. After losing weight, she starts to wear fashionable clothes and her improved body image leads to development of her own edgy style. In contrast to her newfound love of clothes, Josie's circle of friends hasn't changed. She still looks forward to the Friday night dinner out, but for Josie it's what she'll wear and the socializing, not the food, that's most important. Mark's weight loss and improved health lead to thinking more carefully about how he wants to spend his time, and he decides not to return to selling cars. Megan discovers that being a good student is still important to her, but she doesn't feel she's hiding behind the "good student" role anymore. Instead she feels that her life is bigger than being the straight-A student. Joining the softball team and making new friends expands Megan's image of herself. Answer these questions about what has changed for you:

1. What has been the biggest change? _____

_____

2. What change surprised you the most? _____

_____

3. What didn't change? _____

_____

4. Is there anything you would like to change now? _____

_____

REVIEWING YOUR COMPELLING GOAL

It's time to review your compelling goal. Your goal may have changed as you moved through the process of getting WLS and losing weight, or it may have remained the same. It's not uncommon for people to modify or even add to a compelling goal. You may recall that Josie's compelling goal was to resolve her prediabetes and lower her risk of developing diabetes, as her mother did. Mark's compelling goal was to lose enough weight to have a knee replacement and return to work. Megan's compelling goal was to improve her self-esteem and confidence as she launched herself into adulthood. Below, discover how after WLS they meet, revise, or add to their goal.

Compelling Goal Update for Josie, Mark, and Megan

Josie: Josie loses enough weight to resolve her prediabetes. After a challenge with weight regain, she successfully loses and keeps off 65 percent of her excess weight. She enrolls in a two-year business-degree program at her local college and is now focusing on starting an accounting business.

Mark: Mark loses over 70 percent of his excess weight and has both his bad knees replaced. Being able to walk without pain and to feel physically healthy make Mark realize that there are lots of things he wants to do, but returning to selling cars isn't one of them. Mark changes that part of his compelling goal to restoring a 1966 Mustang fastback, maintaining the Mustang club's website, and spending more time with his grandchildren. He takes his grandchild to Disneyland and, without all the extra weight and with new knees, is able to walk around the park and go on rides he would have been excluded from before WLS. It's not surprising that one of the things Mark adds to his list of things he wants to do is start dating. Mark finds that meeting women with the help of an online service increases his confidence, and he hopes to find a woman who enjoys cars as much as he does.

Megan: Megan decides to have WLS the summer after her freshman year at college, and she loses 45 percent of her excess weight with gastric banding. She still struggles with social situations but feels confident enough to try out for her college debate team. Megan's participation in the community softball team leads to several surprises. She finds that she's a powerful hitter and discovers that how much she weighs makes little difference to her team members, who are more interested in how far she can hit the ball and how much fun she is to be around at the postgame parties.

Now it's time to review your compelling goal. Did you reach your goal? Answer these questions about your compelling goal:

1. Did you reach your compelling goal?   ☐ Yes ☐ No

    If not, why not: _____

    If you didn't reach your goal, did you reach part of it?   ☐ Yes ☐ No

    Which part? _____

2. Did your compelling goal change as you lost weight?   ☐ Yes ☐ No

3. If your goal changed, how did it change? _____

---

4. If you reached your compelling goal, what has changed in your life as a result?

5. What hasn't changed? _____

6. Is there a part of your compelling goal you're still working on?   ☐ Yes   ☐ No

   Which part? _____

NEW GOALS

Now it's time to move from WLS and weight loss goals to other life goals. Consider the different parts of your life. What social, occupational, or personal things do you want to do? Was there something you never even thought about doing that you're now thinking about? Is there a challenge you think you might like to take on? At the end of each chapter, we looked at what was next in WLS success. Now it's time for you to decide what's next for your life.

What's Next?

1. *My next life goal is:* _____

   _____

2. *I never thought I would, but now I'm thinking about doing:* _____

   _____

3. *It would be challenging and a risk, but I could:* _____

   _____

Resources

With the increase in WLS rates has come an increase in resources. Check out the following resources to help you with WLS success.

ONLINE WLS RESOURCES (SUPPORT AND INFORMATION)

Weight-loss surgery support groups: Listing of WLS support groups around the United States, wlscenter.com/GroupsInState.htm

National Association for Weight Loss Surgery: Started by a social worker who had WLS; includes a discussion forum, nawls.com

Renewed Reflections: Blog posts by people who have had WLS, including recipes and other good information, www.renewedreflections.com

Obesity Help: Blog postings and online community for people who have had WLS, www.obesityhelp.com

Weight Loss Surgery Channel: A TV network for WLS that has a cool website, www.weightlosssurgerychannel.com

FINDING A SURGEON

American Society for Metabolic and Bariatric Surgery is a professional organization for WLS surgeons and other WLS specialists that can help you find a surgeon: asmbs.org

GENERAL NUTRITIONAL INFORMATION

Standard measurements for healthy portions of specific foods and calorie estimates: www.mypyramid.gov

ELECTRONIC FOOD LOGS

Fitbit: Electronic food logging, online community, www.fitbit.com

The Daily Plate: Electronic food logging, www.thedailyplate.com

PROBLEM EATING

Beck, J. S. 2007. *The Beck Diet Solution: Train Your Brain to Think Like a Thin Person*. Birmingham, AL: Oxmoor House.

Laliberte, M., R. E. McCabe, and V. Taylor. 2009. *The Cognitive Behavioral Workbook for Weight Management*. Oakland, CA: New Harbinger Publications.

Nash, J. D. 1999. *Binge No More: Your Guide to Overcoming Disordered Eating*. Oakland, CA: New Harbinger Publications.

Ross, C. C. 2009. *Binge Eating and Compulsive Overeating Workbook*. Oakland, CA: New Harbinger Publications.

COOKING

Leach, S. M. 2007. *Before and After: Living and Eating Well After Weight-Loss Surgery*. Rev. ed. New York: HarperCollins.

Levine, P., and M. Bontempo-Saray. 2004. *Eating Well After Weight Loss Surgery*. New York: Marlowe and Company.

PSYCHOLOGICAL PROBLEMS

Corcoran, J. 2009. *The Depression Solutions Workbook*. Oakland, CA: New Harbinger Publications.

Marra, T. 2004. *Depressed and Anxious: The Dialectical Behavior Therapy Workbook for Overcoming Depression and Anxiety*. Oakland, CA: New Harbinger Publications.

Silberman, S. A. 2008. *The Insomnia Workbook*. Oakland, CA: New Harbinger Publications.

References

Aasheim, E. T., S. Björkman, T. T. Søvik, M. Engström, S. E. Hanvold, T. Mala, T. Olbers, and T. Bøhmer. 2009. Vitamin status after bariatric surgery: A randomized study of gastric bypass and duodenal switch. *American Journal of Clinical Nutrition* 90 (1):15–22.

Adams, T. D., R. E. Gress, S. C. Smith, R. C. Halverson, S. C. Simper, W. D. Rosamond, M. J. LaMonte, A. M. Stroup, and S. C. Hunt. 2007. Long-term mortality after gastric bypass surgery. *New England Journal of Medicine* 357 (8):753–61.

Aills, L., J. Blankenship, C. Buffington, M. Furtado, and J. Parrott. 2008. ASMBS allied health nutritional guidelines for surgical weight loss patient. *Surgery for Obesity and Related Diseases* 4 (Suppl. 5):S73–108.

American Psychiatric Association (APA). 2000. *Diagnostic and Statistical Manual of Mental Disorders (DSM-IV-TR)*. 4th ed. Text rev. Washington, DC: American Psychiatric Association.

American Society for Metabolic and Bariatric Surgery (ASMBS). 2005. Rationale for surgery: Rationale for the surgical treatment of morbid obesity. www.asbs.org/Newsite07/patients/resources/asbs_rationale.htm

Batsis, J. A., M. M. Clark, K. Grothe, F. Lopez-Jimenez, M. L. Collazo-Clavell, V. K. Somers, and M. G. Sarr. 2009. Self-efficacy after bariatric surgery for obesity: A population-based cohort study. *Appetite* 52 (3):637–45.

Beck, J. S. 2007. *The Beck Diet Solution: Train Your Brain to Think Like a Thin Person*. Birmingham, AL: Oxmoor House.

Berarducci, A. 2007. Bone loss: An emerging problem following obesity surgery. *Orthopaedic Nursing* 26 (5):281–86.

Brolin, R. E., and R. P. Cody. 2008. Weight loss outcome of revisional bariatric operations varies according to the primary procedure. *Annals of Surgery* 248 (2):227–32.

Bueter, M., J. Maroske, A. Thalheimer, M. Gasser, T. Stingl, J. Heimbucher, D. Meyer, K. H. Fuchs, and M. Fein. 2008. Short- and long-term results of laparoscopic gastric banding for morbid obesity. *Langenbeck's Archives of Surgery* 393 (2):199–205.

Carels, R. A., L. A. Darby, S. Rydin, O. M. Douglass, H. M. Cacciapaglia, and W. H. O'Brien. 2005. The relationship between self-monitoring, outcome expectancies, difficulties with eating and exercise, and physical activity and weight loss treatment outcomes. *Annals of Behavioral Medicine* 30 (3):182–90.

Cash, T. F. 1997. *The Body Image Workbook: An 8-Step Program for Learning to Like Your Looks.* Oakland, CA: New Harbinger Publications.

Dalla Paola, L., and E. Faglia. 2006. Treatment of diabetic foot ulcer: An overview of strategies for clinical approach. *Current Diabetes Reviews* 2 (4):431–47.

Fontaine, K. R., D. T. Redden, C. Wang, A. O. Westfall, and D. B. Allison. 2003. Years of life lost due to obesity. *Journal of the American Medical Association* 289 (2):187–93.

Friedman, K. E., J. A. Ashmore, and K. L. Applegate. 2008. Recent experiences of weight-based stigmatization in a weight loss surgery population: Psychological and behavioral correlates. *Obesity* 16 (Suppl. 2):S69–74.

Gómez, V., T. S. Riall, and G. A. Gómez. 2008. Outcomes in bariatric surgery in the older patient population in Texas. *Journal of Surgical Research* 147 (2):270–75.

Grilo, C. M., M. A. White, R. M. Masheb, B. S. Rothschild, and C. H. Burke-Martindale. 2006. Relation of childhood sexual abuse and other forms of maltreatment to 12-month postoperative outcomes in extremely obese gastric bypass patients. *Obesity Surgery* 16 (4):454–60.

Guth, E. S., and E. H. Livingston. 2008. Bariatric surgery: Is it right for your patient? *Postgraduate Medicine* 120 (3):1–13.

Heinberg, L. J., K. Keating, and L. Simonelli. 2010. Discrepancy between ideal and realistic goal weights in three bariatric procedures: Who is likely to be unrealistic? *Obesity Surgery* 20 (2):148–53.

Hinojosa, M. W., J. E. Varela, D. Parikh, B. R. Smith, X. M. Nguyen, and N. T. Nguyen. 2009. National trends in use and outcome of laparoscopic adjustable gastric banding. *Surgery for Obesity and Related Diseases* 5 (2):150–55.

Howell, M. J., C. H. Schenck, and S. J. Crow. 2009. A review of nighttime eating disorders. *Sleep Medicine Reviews* 13 (1):23–34.

Kaly, P., S. Orellana, T. Torrella, C. Takagishi, L. Saff-Koche, and M. M. Murr. 2008. Unrealistic weight loss expectations in candidates for bariatric surgery. *Surgery for Obesity and Related Diseases* 4 (1):6–10.

Karlsson, J., C. Taft, A. Rydén, L. Sjöström, and M. Sullivan. 2007. Ten-year trends in health-related quality of life after surgical and conventional treatment for severe obesity: The SOS intervention study. *International Journal of Obesity* 31 (8):1248–61.

Kim, R. J., J. M. Langer, A. W. Baker, D. E. Filter, N. N. Williams, and D. B. Sarwer. 2008. Psychosocial status in adolescents undergoing bariatric surgery. *Obesity Surgery* 18 (1):27–33.

Kurian, M. S., B. Thompson, and B. K. Davidson. 2005. *Weight Loss Surgery for Dummies*. Hoboken, NJ: Wiley Publishing.

Lakdawala, M. A., A. Bhasker, D. Mulchandani, S. Goel, and S. Jain. 2010. Comparison between the results of laparoscopic sleeve gastrectomy and laparoscopic Roux-en-Y gastric bypass in the Indian population: A retrospective 1-year study. *Obesity Surgery* 20 (1):1–6.

Longitudinal Assessment of Bariatric Surgery (LABS) Consortium. 2009. Perioperative safety in the longitudinal assessment of bariatric surgery. *New England Journal of Medicine* 361 (5):445–54.

Madan, A. K., D. S. Tichansky, and R. J. Taddeucci. 2007. Postoperative laparoscopic bariatric surgery patients do not remember potential complications. *Obesity Surgery* 17 (7):885–88.

Marsk, R., E. Jonas, H. Gartzios, D. Stockeld, L. Granström, and J. Freedman. 2009. High revision rates after laparoscopic vertical banded gastroplasty. *Surgery for Obesity and Related Diseases* 5 (1):94–98.

Mason, E. E., K. E. Renquist, W. Zhang, IBSR Data Contributors. 2003. Trends in bariatric surgery, 1986–2001. *Obesity Surgery* 13:225.

Moizé, V. L., X. Pi-Sunyer, H. Mochari, and J. Vidal. 2010. Nutritional pyramid for post-gastric bypass patients. *Obesity Surgery* 20 (8):1133–41.

Nishimura, S., I. Manabe, and R. Nagai. 2009. Adipose tissue inflammation in obesity and metabolic syndrome. *Discovery Medicine* 8 (41):55–60.

Norris, L. 2007. Psychiatric issues in bariatric surgery. *Psychiatric Clinics of North America* 30 (4):717–38.

O'Brien, P. E., S. M. Sawyer, C. Laurie, W. A. Brown, S. Skinner, F. Veit, et al. 2010. Laparoscopic adjustable gastric banding in severely obese adolescents: A randomized trial. *Journal of the American Medical Association* 303 (6):519–26.

Pollack, A. 2010. Panel votes to expand surgery for less obese. The *New York Times*, December 4, B1.

Potoczna, N., S. Harfmann, R. Steffen, R. Briggs, N. Bieri, and F. Horber. 2008. Bowel habits after bariatric surgery. *Obesity Surgery* 18 (10):1287–96.

Pratt, J. S., C. M. Lenders, E. A. Dionne, A. G. Hoppin, G. L. Hsu, T. H. Inge, et al. 2009. Best practice updates for pediatric/adolescent weight loss surgery. *Obesity* 17 (5):901–10.

Robinson, M. K. 2009. Surgical treatment of obesity: Weighing the facts. *New England Journal of Medicine* 361 (5):520–21.

Sarwer, D. B., J. K. Thompson, J. E. Mitchell, and J. P. Rubin. 2008a. Psychological considerations of the bariatric surgery patient undergoing body-contouring surgery. *Plastic and Reconstructive Surgery* 121 (6):423e–34e.

Sarwer, D. B., T. A. Wadden, R. H. Moore, A. W. Baker, L. M. Gibbons, S. E. Raper, and N. N. Williams. 2008b. Preoperative eating behavior, postoperative dietary adherence, and weight loss after gastric bypass surgery. *Surgery for Obesity and Related Diseases* 4 (5):640–46.

Shah, M., V. Simha, and A. Garg. 2006. Review: Long-term impact of bariatric surgery on body weight, comorbidities, and nutritional status. *Journal of Clinical Endocrinology and Metabolism* 91 (11):4223–31.

Song, Z., K. Reinhardt, M. Buzdon, and P. Liao. 2008. Association between support group attendance and weight loss after Roux-en-Y gastric bypass. *Surgery for Obesity and Related Diseases* 4 (2):1000–1003.

Strain, G. W., M. Gagner, A. Pomp, G. Dakin, W. B. Inabnet, J. Hsieh, L. Heacock, and P. Christos. 2009. Comparison of weight loss and body composition changes with four surgical procedures. *Surgery for Obesity and Related Diseases* 5 (5):582–87.

Tice, J. A., L. Karliner, J. Walsh, A. J. Petersen, and M. D. Feldman. 2008. Gastric banding or bypass? A systematic review comparing the two most popular bariatric procedures. *American Journal of Medicine* 121 (10):885–93.

Topart, P., G. Becouarn, and P. Ritz. 2007. Biliopancreatic diversion with duodenal switch or gastric bypass for failed gastric banding: Retrospective study from two institutions with preliminary results. *Surgery for Obesity and Related Diseases* 3 (5):521–25.

Van der Beek, E. S., W. Te Riele, T. F. Specken, D. Boerma, and B. van Ramshorst. 2010. The impact of reconstructive procedures following bariatric surgery on patient well-being and quality of life. *Obesity Surgery* 20 (1):36–41.

Welch, G., C. Wesolowski, S. Zagarins, J. Kuhn, J. Romanelli, J. Garb, and N. Allen. 2010. Evaluation of clinical outcomes for gastric bypass surgery: Results from a comprehensive follow-up study. *Obesity Surgery.* doi: 10.1007/s11695-009-0069-3.

Wittgrove, A. C., and T. Martinez. 2009. Laparoscopic gastric bypass in patients 60 years and older: Early postoperative morbidity and resolution of comorbidities. *Obesity Surgery* 19 (11):1472–76.

Xanthakos, S. A. 2008. Bariatric surgery for extreme adolescent obesity: Indications, outcomes, and physiologic effects on the gut-brain axis. *Pathophysiology* 15 (2):135–46.

Zeller, M. H., A. V. Modi, J. G. Noll, J. D. Long, and T. H. Inge. 2009. Psychosocial functioning improves following adolescent bariatric surgery. *Obesity* 17 (5):985–90.

Doreen A. Samelson, Ed.D., MSCP, is a medical psychologist specializing in weight loss surgery and the treatment of eating disorders. She is committed to helping people with weight or food-related problems experience improved health and quality of life. An experienced public speaker, she regularly lectures on weight and food-related topics, and is author of *Feeding the Starving Mind*. She lives in northern California.

Foreword writer **Arnold D. Salzberg, MD,** is a member of the surgical faculty at the University of California, San Francisco. He specializes in laparoscopic high risk weight loss surgery, liver surgery, and surgery on those with end stage renal disease and transplants. He has researched surgical advanced technology at Stanford University and high-risk bariatric surgery at the University of California, San Francisco.

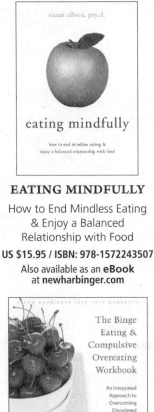
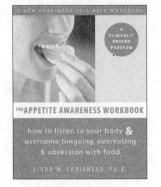
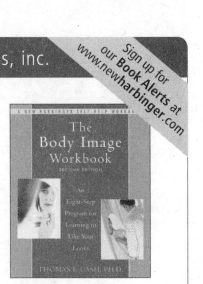
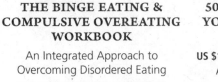
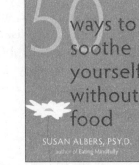
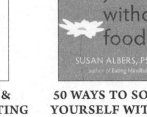
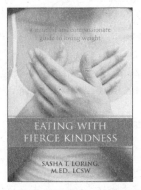